Living Your Life with Car through Acceptance and Commitment Therapy

This valuable self-help book for people affected by cancer, their loved ones and friends focuses on self-care when life hurts. It explores the impact of cancer and explains why the usual ways of coping may leave people stuck.

The first book of its kind to focus on the scientifically based Acceptance and Commitment Therapy (ACT) approach, it helps people to find ways to cope with painful thoughts and feelings, and to rebuild a meaningful life despite the cancer. With an emphasis on value-based living the book illustrates skills such as mindfulness and the development of acceptance to help people affected by cancer to participate in a fuller life and gain a greater sense of well-being. It combines evidence-based practice with the experiences of people who are living with cancer in the form of numerous quotations throughout, as well as paper and pencil 'thought' exercises.

Living Your Life with Cancer through Acceptance and Commitment Therapy helps people affected by cancer to feel more able to sit with the uncertainty of their future, show themselves kindness and compassion and to learn to be true to themselves, no matter what the cancer throws at them. It is also important reading for psychological therapists working in oncology.

Anne Johnson is a Consultant Clinical Psychologist who has worked in cancer and palliative care with adults and children in the NHS.

Claire Delduca is a Principal Clinical Psychologist who has worked within specialist cancer and palliative care services for adults in the NHS for seven years.

Reg Morris is a Consultant Clinical Psychologist and director of clinical psychology training who has worked therapeutically and researched with people affected by long-term conditions since 1995.

About the artist:

Mark Harvey, an artist and illustrator originating from Southampton, provided the illustrations displayed in this book.

Living Your Life with Cancer through Acceptance and Commitment Therapy

Flying over Thunderstorms

Anne Johnson
Claire Delduca
and Reg Morris

Illustrations by
Mark Harvey

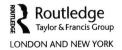
Routledge
Taylor & Francis Group
LONDON AND NEW YORK

First published 2021
by Routledge
2 Park Square, Milton Park, Abingdon, Oxon OX14 4RN

and by Routledge
605 Third Avenue, New York, NY 10158

Routledge is an imprint of the Taylor & Francis Group, an informa business

British Library Cataloguing-in-Publication Data
A catalogue record for this book is available from the British Library

Library of Congress Cataloging-in-Publication Data
Names: Johnson, Anne (Consultant clinical psychologist), author.
Title: Living your life with cancer: an ACT approach: flying over thunderstorms/Anne Johnson, Claire Delduca and Reg Morris.
Description: Milton Park, Abingdon, Oxon; New York: Routledge, 2021. | Includes bibliographical references and index.
Identifiers: LCCN 2020056915 (print) | LCCN 2020056916 (ebook) | ISBN 9780367549237 (hardback) | ISBN 9780367549244 (paperback) | ISBN 9781003091202 (ebook)
Subjects: LCSH: Cancer–Patients–Psychology. | Acceptance and commitment therapy.
Classification: LCC RC262 .J62 2021 (print) | LCC RC262 (ebook) | DDC 616.99/40651–dc23
LC record available at https://lccn.loc.gov/2020056915
LC ebook record available at https://lccn.loc.gov/2020056916

ISBN: 978-0-367-54923-7 (hbk)
ISBN: 978-0-367-54924-4 (pbk)
ISBN: 978-1-003-09120-2 (ebk)

Typeset in Univers
by Deanta Global Publishing Services, Chennai, India

Access the Support Material: www.routledge.com/9780367549244

Dedication

This book is dedicated to our loving families and dearest friends who have laughed with us, cried with us, kept us going and flown with us over our own thunderstorms to enable us to realize our ambition of writing this book.

For Charlie, Bella, Sienna and Liz.

Contents

Foreword

Lynda Thomas- Chief Executive, Macmillan Cancer Support

It's no exaggeration to say being diagnosed with cancer can be devastating. Nothing can prepare someone for hearing the dreaded 'C word' for the first time. It can turn a person's life upside down and is life-changing in many different, and often unexpected, ways.

Sadly, it's a traumatic experience one in two of us will go through, and currently nearly three million people in the UK are living with cancer. By 2030, this figure is projected to reach four million.

More people than ever need support. Which is why, as Chief Executive of Macmillan Cancer Support, I feel privileged and humbled to lead one of the UK's biggest charities – one that touched the lives of 8.3 million people affected by cancer in 2019.

I am also honored to have been given the opportunity to write the foreword for this book, which I believe will be a great addition to the resources for people living with cancer and health professionals.

There is no 'one size fits all' approach when it comes to cancer and treatment. Cancer affects everyone differently and while the physical effects can be life-altering, it impacts people's emotional well-being and mental health too.

It is common for people to report experiencing difficult thoughts and feel a loss of control. There is often a societal pressure felt by many to put on a 'brave face' and be 'positive'. Even after finishing treatment, anxiety can still leave people feeling overwhelmed, and often the impact of cancer continues long after treatment is completed.

Macmillan's fundamental aim is to help people live as fully as they can. For this to happen, a person's holistic needs must be considered. This is where methods like the Acceptance and Commitment Therapy (ACT) explored within the upcoming chapters, come in.

People living with cancer, many of whom along with their families have input their voices and thoughts into this book, often report fears and concerns about the future, and how their illness will affect their families too.

ACT is designed to provide the tools and understanding to enable people living with cancer and their families to feel they have more choice over what they do, while learning how to be more flexible in their approach to painful thoughts, images, feelings, sensations, memories or situations. It's important to acknowledge difficult thoughts and feelings, rather than avoid them – freeing up precious time and energy to focus on other things.

The exercises also aim to equip people with extra tools to help recognize thoughts and feelings as just that, and to help the reader feel more able to choose to do what works best for them rather than what is expected, no matter what cancer throws at them.

This book has clear and simple coping strategies that could help you to look after yourself when things are tough, and skills and resources are included to support psychological well-being during treatment, after treatment and for those in palliative care.

Additionally, it's important to note not that it's not just those diagnosed who are affected. Family and friends often struggle with feelings of helplessness, and it's often hard to know what to say, which is why understanding the coping strategies in this book can be beneficial for both patients and their loved ones.

Two of the authors of this book have worked as Macmillan Clinical Psychologists. Dr. Claire Delduca and Dr. Anne Johnson have supported both children and adults coping with the impact of cancer for over 25 years. There are over 12,000 Macmillan professionals working across the UK and they are employed by a range of partner organizations, all delivering and developing services in Macmillan's name.

It's dedicated professionals like these who enabled Macmillan to provide an estimated 1.9 million people last year with in-depth, personal support.

With 1,000 people a day diagnosed with cancer, it's reassuring there are so many professionals out there prepared to go that extra mile to support people as they navigate their way through what may be an extremely traumatic time.

It's also heartening to see our own Macmillan professionals producing resources like this book which can be read by anyone with cancer who wants tools and advice on what they can do to live life as fully as possible.

Preface

When we began working with people affected by serious health conditions like cancer, we heard many of them telling us that they had strong and worrying thoughts, such as "Will the treatment work?", "Am I going to die?" and "How are my family going to cope?". They felt immense pain and loss as they may no longer be able to fulfill their hopes, ambitions and dreams for their futures. They were filled with painful but understandable feelings of uncertainty about almost all aspects of their lives going forward. This pain and loss was felt not only by the people who had been given the diagnosis, but also by their partners, children, other relatives, friends, colleagues, neighbors and even the professionals working with them.

We quickly noticed that more traditional approaches to therapy, such as Cognitive Behavioral Therapy (CBT), often did not fit the needs of the people we were working with. Focusing upon challenging and changing 'unhelpful' or 'irrational' thoughts or reducing distress often unintentionally implied the wrong message. How could people who were facing some of the most difficult and scary challenges in their lives find ways to feel happier or less upset about the situation they found themselves in? A situation that they did not choose? Thoughts and feelings that they just could not change or control?

This was highlighted even further when we listened to people who had been given a palliative diagnosis or short prognosis. They were facing the prospect of having less time than they had hoped and were often limited by pain, physical changes and significant fatigue. They were facing the end of their lives and making incredibly difficult decisions about whether to have more treatment (but possibly risking feeling more unwell) or to step away from treatment to prioritize the (possibly shorter) time they had doing the things that mattered most to them, such as seeing their loved ones. We felt privileged to be able to hear their stories and to be with these people during those most painful times.

We were also struck by how many people came to us who were hugely resourceful and resilient. People who had got themselves through many challenges in their lives but were left feeling floored by cancer. They often felt helpless and hopeless; struggling to understand why they had the cancer, why they didn't feel as though they could cope this time, why they couldn't get rid of their painful thoughts and feelings or why they didn't feel lucky, grateful or happier as there were "always people worse off than me!".

We had begun to be interested in Acceptance and Commitment Therapy and had attended training with Russ Harris. Hearing these stories strongly supported the need for us to use a therapeutic approach that validated people's experiences – one that helped people to learn about and understand that difficult thoughts and feelings were 'normal' and important. The thoughts and feelings were more often than not telling people that there were things in their life that they cared greatly for. That the gap between what they had hoped for in their lives and where they were now felt large. An ACT approach focuses upon acknowledging and allowing (rather than challenging) painful thoughts and feelings. It promotes a 'flexible' response to distress, based upon reconnecting to your values and 'doing' what works.

The ACT approach helped people to understand why their usual ways of coping were no longer working. This was not because they were not trying hard enough or because they were failing in some way, but because as humans we naturally feel pain at times and all too often life is tough. We found that ACT helped people affected by cancer to feel more able to sit with the uncertainty of their future, show themselves kindness and compassion and to learn to be true to themselves, no matter what the cancer threw at them.

We noticed that ACT frees people from the tyranny of 'positive' thinking, such as:

● The futility of cultural beliefs, such as 'don't give up the fight'.

● The 'battle' language which surrounds cancer, which implies that people should be 'strong' or 'brave' or 'warriors'.

● Or the assumption that cancer is a 'journey' with an end point that people should aim for which is 'happy' or free of pain, suffering and long-term difficulties.

Using this approach over the years has transformed our clinical practice. We have had the privilege to witness some of the most poignant, deeply touching and meaningful changes that people have made. Changes which have brought meaning, connection and fulfillment to the lives of these people, even in the face of great pain, sadness and loss. These experiences still touch us strongly and will stay with us throughout our careers.

The stories and changes that we have witnessed people making when life is at its most painful have enabled us to make changes to our own lives too. We have learned to recognize what really matters to us and this has shown us the importance of not taking for granted the people and things that matter most to us in our lives. In essence, we have personally experienced the powerful difference that an ACT approach can offer too.

Writing this book has been an ambition of ours for a long time. We wanted to write a book to share our model of ACT for people affected by cancer, in the same way that ACT has been shared with people with other serious health conditions. This model and book are based upon the writing of esteemed clinicians who we have had the privilege of being supported by, inspiring training we have attended, experiences which have been shared by our respected colleagues and most importantly the stories, feedback and perspectives of the people we have worked with. The process of writing this book has taken a long time. It has been both rewarding and painful, but to us it always felt worthwhile and it mattered. We hope that this book can make a difference to you, however you have been affected by the impact of cancer. Thank you for taking some of your precious time to read it.

Acknowledgments

The authors gratefully acknowledge Russ Harris and Dr. Ray Owen for permitting them to adapt and use some of the ACT-based exercises they developed.

Russ and Ray have both been and continue to be inspirations in our clinical practice of ACT. We thank them both for their contributions to this book. We are proud that they have both been kind enough to support us with the process.

We want to thank all the people who gave us permission to use their voices throughout this book. You have helped to shape the book and most importantly to bring it to life.

We also want to thank the people who have been affected by cancer we have worked with over the years. It has been a privilege to work with and learn from you as you have shared your experiences with us. You have inspired us to write this book to share our learning and to connect with others further afield.

Thanks to Kat Fitzgerald, who guided and led us in developing our first ACT-based group, as our interest in ACT for cancer was first sparking.

Thanks also to Emma Keenan, who took the time to share the book with people who have been affected by cancer and to gather the feedback we needed to make the book helpful and usable.

To Dr. Victoria Samuel, we thank you for the time you have taken to steer us back onto the right track when we had lost our way.

Our heartfelt thanks goes to Julie Armytage, who allowed us to use her caramel voice for the audio exercises which accompany the book. She, Kate Morgan and the team at Velindre Cancer Center held our hands and fed us cake through many highs and lows along the way.

To Mark Harvey, thank you for the time you have taken to create the illustrations to bring color and vibrancy to the book.

To our family and friends, who shared their love and support and read over many drafts for us. And thank you and love to our partners and children, who kept us going, helped us through and gave us the hugs we needed to get over our own thunderstorms on this journey to a book that we hope will matter to you as much as it matters to us.

PART
1 Understanding the impact of cancer

"The word cancer turned my life upside down. I felt like everything I love was suddenly being thrown out the window. I was devastated, I couldn't believe it was true ... what did it mean for me, my family and my future?"

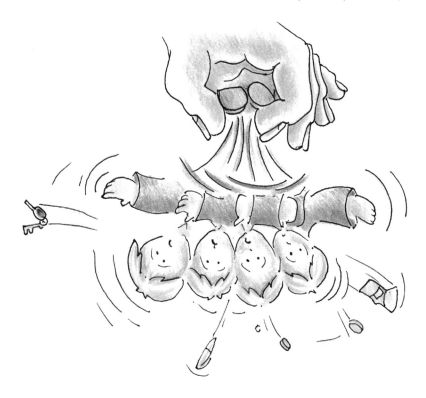

About this book

This book has been written by psychologists working with people who are living with the impact of cancer. It is based upon information, ideas and strategies that people who have experienced cancer, along with their family, friends and professionals, have found useful. The framework for this book is an approach called Acceptance and Commitment Therapy (ACT).

The book describes the kinds of changes that can occur after a diagnosis of cancer. Often, the physical effects of cancer are the most visibly obvious changes that people are faced with. These can include changes to your body – such as hair loss, weight change and scarring. You may experience changes to your appetite. You may also experience other problems like nausea, fatigue and pain.

"As I left hospital and rested for a few weeks, body image started to become an issue for me. Every time I looked in the mirror, I despised what greeted me, a disfigured old looking guy ... a worried looking guy".

In addition to physical changes, there are the psychological effects of cancer that can be difficult to deal with. These may include:

● Understanding what is happening to you.

● Worrying about the treatment and whether it will work.

● Feeling uncertain about what is going to happen in the future for you and your family.

● Worries about dying.

● Adjusting to changes in your body, identity and life.

● Feelings of loss about important roles, plans and hopes.

● Feelings of sadness that things are not the same as they were before.

It can feel like your thoughts and feelings take over. Many people feel like they are struggling at times or are just not able to be themselves anymore.

This book aims to help you cope with some of the psychological, physical and relationship changes that can happen following a diagnosis of cancer.

It hopes to help you understand:

● What you are doing that is working well.

● What you are doing that is not working so well.

● What to do at times when you are feeling stuck or lost.

● What to do to be the person you want to be and to rebuild your life after a cancer diagnosis.

(Note: it is important to note early on that if you have any concerns about symptoms, side-effects of treatment or how you are feeling physically, always seek advice from your medical team. You can request psychological support from your care provider or GP if you feel unable to cope with the emotional impact of the cancer on your own. If you are really struggling and feel unable to keep yourself safe, there are crisis support service details in Part 4 of this book).

Who is this book for?

The book is for anyone affected by a diagnosis of cancer. This might include:

● The person who has had a diagnosis of cancer.

● Family, friends and carers.

● Anyone working with someone who has had a cancer diagnosis.

We know that many people can be affected by cancer in their lives and in different ways.

You may be the person who has been given a diagnosis of cancer, either recently or a long time ago. There could be many worries and fears showing up. These could be about what you are facing now, about how your future will be affected or if you will get through it. You may feel overwhelmed, numb or even grateful that the cancer was found. You may feel very disconnected from the life and future you hoped to have. It could be that you feel as though there is no hope at all. Perhaps life feels very similar and you feel OK. A whole variety of feelings often arise at different (and sometimes unexpected) times. Many people try to hide or 'bottle up' their feelings from their loved ones in order to try to protect them from more distress and worry. Or because they worry that people will think they are not coping.

Alternatively, it could be that you are a person who is supporting or worried about a loved one who has had a diagnosis of cancer. You may be a parent, child, other relative or friend. You may be worried about how you are going to look after them, frightened that you are going to lose them or upset that your relationship has changed. People who are living with, caring for or close to the person who has been given the diagnosis also often feel unable to talk about their feelings or ask for help. However, you are living with the impact of cancer too.

You may also be a professional who is interested in learning more about the impact of cancer to help you to support the people you work with. This may be a new area for you or you may have many years of experience to draw on.

We hope that this book is helpful for everyone who is living or working with the impact of cancer.

"It's like a rollercoaster, just when you think you've got the hang of it you've got another big dip. It takes time to get used to the ups and downs of life after a diagnosis of cancer".

"Cancer changed my life. At the beginning it changed my life for the worse – it scared me, hurt me, made me feel vulnerable and lost".

The impact of cancer

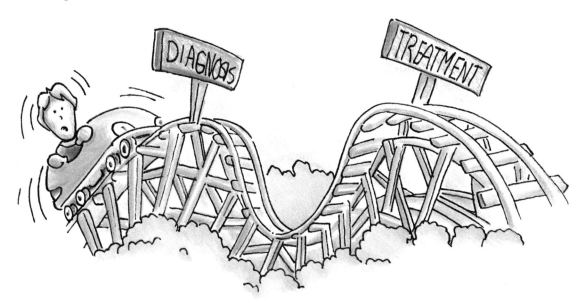

Throughout the book, we will use phrases such as "after a diagnosis of cancer", "affected by cancer" or "living with the impact of cancer". This is to represent the impact that a cancer diagnosis can have both in the short term, as well as the longer term. This is for the person who has been given the diagnosis and for those around them.

Importantly, we have chosen not to specifically distinguish between different diagnoses, stages of cancer or prognoses within this book. This is because we have chosen to use an approach that most people we have worked with have found helpful, regardless of the type or stage of the cancer, their treatment plan or the outcome.

People have found this approach helpful when they:

● Have been diagnosed with an early-stage cancer.

● Are undergoing treatment.

● Are in a monitoring or follow up phase.

● Have been given a palliative diagnosis.

● Are facing the end of their life.

● Are supporting someone who has experienced cancer.

Therefore, whatever your experience of cancer and however it has affected you, we hope this book will enable you to understand your difficult thoughts and feelings, look after yourself and to make decisions that are right for you. As well as to help you to be who you want to be and to find fulfillment and meaning, even when life hurts.

Acceptance and Commitment Therapy (ACT) and cancer

The approach that we use within this book is based upon a framework called Acceptance and Commitment Therapy (more commonly known as ACT). A key message of ACT and this book is that it is normal to experience difficult thoughts and feelings. Our usual ways of dealing with problems and distress may not work, especially after a difficult life event like a diagnosis of cancer. In fact, they may at times make you feel worse. This book aims to help you explore ACT-based ideas and to consider if these could help you when you are living with the impact of cancer. We hope the ideas in this book help you to think about what works best for you and to give you extra tools to use through difficult times. It may help you to think about what you can do to move forward in your life.

"Cancer has focused my view on what really matters to me in life and has given me a sense of control over what I can do to live well today and in my future".

"I've gone from being a well person who feels in control of my life and my future to facing the unknown with no road map. I just want to get back to being me".

What you will find in this book

After receiving a diagnosis of cancer, you may feel overwhelmed and as though you are unable to take in a lot of information. You might find the idea of reading this book all in one go too difficult. It could be helpful to read small bits at a time and come back to it. To make this easier, the book is split into sections so that you can find the information relevant to you when you need it. Real life examples and quotes from people affected by cancer are included throughout the book.

The book has four main parts:

Part 1: Understanding the impact of cancer on your life

The first part of this book describes why we have written the book and explains the approach of the book. It focuses upon helping you to understand the psychological impact of cancer, using an ACT framework. It explains why your usual ways of coping may no longer be working for you and helps you to consider if it could be helpful for you to add new tools into your coping toolkit.

Part 2: Living a meaningful life after a diagnosis of cancer

Part 2 has three sections. They describe things you can do to recognize difficult thoughts and feelings and to look after yourself when they come up. It also gives ideas that could help you to live your life and do the things that matter when painful things, such as feelings of uncertainty about your future, show up. This part of the book aims to help you to lead a fulfilling life, despite a cancer diagnosis.

Part 3: Looking after yourself

Part 3 focuses on the importance of self-care when you have been affected by cancer. It explores some practical strategies you could use as well as some ideas that can help with common problems associated with cancer, such as sleep, pain, fatigue and eating difficulties. It aims to help to remind you of the importance of looking after your mind and body to boost your overall well-being.

Part 4: Moving forward

The last section brings together and summarizes what the book has covered. It aims to help you to think about which of the new skills you would like to hold on to and how you can continue to build on the things you have learned. It helps you to consider how you can care for yourself physically and emotionally going forward, as you reconnect to a sense of meaning and purpose in your life.

The tools of this book

There are a number of symbols and 'tools' which will help you navigate and use this book. All the sections of the book include the following:

Quotes	You will find quotes and stories from people affected by cancer written in blue throughout the book.
	There are 'key messages' summaries at the end of different sections throughout the book.
	There are several exercises that you can try throughout the book.
	There are several audio recordings of exercises that you can find on the linked website. The link to the website is on page ? of this book.

A quick note

Some of the information in the book may not be what you expect. You may worry that you will feel anxious or upset if you spend time thinking about your situation. We hope that the book will help give you new ways of coping with these thoughts and feelings. If at any point you feel overwhelmed, try the 'dropping anchor' exercise in Part 2.

 KEY MESSAGES

● This book is for everyone affected by cancer, including family, friends and professionals.

● It has been written to help you to understand and cope with the impact of cancer in your life using ACT.

● This book uses an ACT-informed approach to help you to recognize what you do that is helpful or unhelpful in taking you toward a life that works for you.

● It will also give ideas of new things that you may want to try.

● The book intends to help you to recognize what matters to you in your life and to do things that take you toward this.

Introduction – the psychological impact of cancer

Nothing can prepare you for the shock of first hearing the words, "it's CANCER". Feelings such as fear, anxiety, hope, anger, guilt and sadness may threaten to overwhelm you. Before you have a chance to catch your breath, you may find your mind rushing. Your mind is trying to make sense of how you have got to this point, what has happened and what that may mean for you, your family and your life going forward. Many people who have been diagnosed with cancer feel worried or uncertain about their future. This can happen as soon as they are diagnosed, as well as during treatment and at any point afterward. Over time, other feelings may also arise, including low mood (or depression), loss, feeling out of control or hopelessness and helplessness.

> "We finally left the hospital and somehow made our way to a coffee shop … I was a wreck, fidgeting on my feet, occupying my hands with whatever I could find, wiping tear after tear away from my cheeks as I waited for my wife to come back to the table".

> "The world kept going on around me in a blur… my mind was so stuck trying to understand what was going on that I couldn't focus. Why me? Why now? … I couldn't find an answer".

When you are affected by cancer, you may also be dealing with many other difficulties or changes at the same time. You are likely to be coping with the impact of the treatment on your body – such as feeling sick or tired, being in pain, experiencing sleep problems or losing your hair. Many people find that they struggle to eat during and after treatment too. You may have difficulties with thinking, such as concentration and memory problems or 'chemobrain'. Sometimes these things can last for a long time after treatment has finished.

It could be that you find it more difficult to do things that you used to do every day, such as looking after yourself or your family, being out with friends, taking part in your hobbies and staying active. You may not be able to work and have stressful practical concerns, such as how to pay your bills. All these difficulties add to the emotional burden that you are facing.

> "I'm usually not a worrier, but once I had my diagnosis I thought "if I can get cancer, what else can happen?", "will it get worse?", "will the treatment work?", "how will I know if it has come back or not?" or "how long will I live?". "I felt like I'd lost control".

> "I wanted to get back to how I was before the cancer. That was my aim and what kept me going. My depression came from the fact I'd never be quite the same as I was. I put myself under too much pressure to get back to how I was. It's important to realize there will not just be physical changes but mental changes as well and your body has gone through a lot".

> "The thoughts just kept going on and on in my head. I thought I was going mad".

Partners, family members or friends also often feel worried, frightened and overwhelmed by the diagnosis and treatment, as well as the longer-term impact it has on their loved one(s) and themselves. They frequently worry about things like what will happen, how they will look after their loved one, what to say and how they or the family will manage. They often notice if their loved one is struggling, even if this isn't obvious and try to help in any way they can. This means that they may also find that their role in the relationship or family changes which can be challenging to adjust to.

> "My husband was so ill during chemotherapy that I needed to do everything for the kids and in the house, as well as look after him … I was exhausted and couldn't moan to him … it wasn't his fault … I felt alone".

> "I had to give up work to look after my mum during her radiotherapy, she needed to be at the hospital everyday … I missed seeing my work colleagues and felt so sad, cross and overwhelmed … don't get me wrong, I wanted to be there for her, but it was hard".

Life may look very different to how it did before the diagnosis and treatment. The gap between where you are in reality and where you want to be in your life can feel big. This gap can continue for many years after treatment, even if professionals tell you that you or your loved one are 'cancer free'. People could be telling you to think positively, saying you are lucky and should be happy. However, you may feel as though you are still facing an uncertain future, which is scary and threatening.

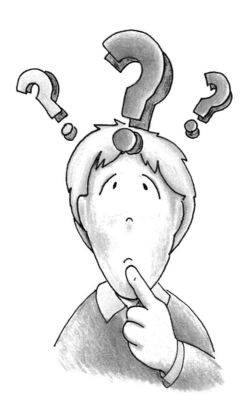

So, when you or someone you care about has been diagnosed with cancer you can face two huge challenges or threats:

1. How to deal with the practical challenges of the illness and treatment.
2. How to cope with all sorts of upsetting thoughts and feelings.

The fight / flight / freeze mechanism

As humans, our usual way to react to threats is with our innate 'fight, flight or freeze' system. This is a survival mechanism that has been passed down by our ancestors over thousands of years. In fact, we can think back to our cave people ancestors and how they would react to a potential threat to help us better understand this system.

Imagine the scene: a cave person is out hunting or gathering for dinner. They reach a clearing when they hear rustling in the nearby leaves. A saber-toothed tiger suddenly jumps in front of them. In this moment, they experience a range of unpleasant emotions (such as fear, panic, anger). Despite how they are feeling, it is likely that what they do next will happen without them thinking too much about it – they will react 'automatically'. To stay safe, the cave person will do one of the following:

- Attack the tiger before it hurts them (fight).

- Run away from the tiger to a place of safety (flight).

- Stay very still until the tiger has gone (freeze).

- Faint or drop to the floor and play dead (severe freeze).

In a similar way to the tiger jumping out in front of the cave person, cancer may have stopped you in your tracks. You may have felt scared, anxious, angry, hopeless, helpless or any number of other painful emotions. Your automatic reaction could be to:

- Do anything you can to get rid of the cancer (fight)

    "I kept having chemotherapy even when I felt so sick".

- Try to remove yourself or escape from the situation (flight)

    "I avoided friends who wanted to talk about my treatment".

- Pretend the situation is not happening (freeze)

    "I found another lump and just couldn't face it; I would avoid touching it and didn't tell anyone".

- Shut down and withdraw from the world (severe freeze)

    "I just couldn't feel anything anymore; I just went to bed and slept".

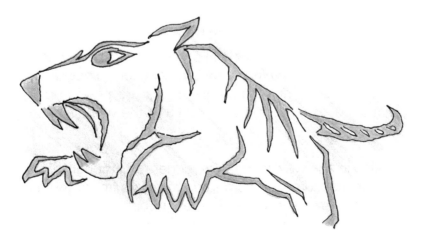

Beyond fight / flight / freeze – our minds as a survival mechanism

Once the immediate threat has gone and the cave person returns home to safety, they might think about what happened and how they could have prevented the tiger attack. They might consider whether it is safe to return to that clearing. They could worry whether the tiger will come again or whether there will be more tigers around next time they leave the camp. They might think about what they can do differently to reduce their risk of harm if the tiger were to come back and what they can do to protect their tribe from a tiger attack.

After a diagnosis of cancer, you may find yourself worrying about the past and the future. You may also find yourself thinking about the past, trying to understand why you or your loved one got cancer, what went wrong and if there was anyone to blame? You may worry about how you will cope with treatment, what you can do to stop it coming back and keep checking to see if it has gone.

> "When I was diagnosed with cancer, I kept thinking 'Why me? What did I do?' I was desperate to know why … because if I did, I stood a chance of stopping it coming back … my mind went crazy spinning in circles".

> "Every time the letter came through the door for my check-up scan … my mind went into overdrive … . Will it be back? … Am I OK? … I would obsessively check my body for any signs, aches, pains, lumps … I was a mess".

When something particularly stressful or traumatic has happened, like a cancer diagnosis, you can become more hyper-vigilant to any threats – you may find yourself worrying more about other bad things happening to yourself or others. You may find yourself being more alert to danger in situations. Now you are aware of the threat and that it is 'real', your mind is primed to stay on high alert and do everything it can to keep you safe.

Our minds are the most successful survival mechanism that human beings have. Our minds have evolved to rapidly notice and react to danger in order to protect us. They use information from previous similar experiences to problem-solve, predict the 'worst-case scenario' and then develop a plan to deal with the potential threats – to get rid of or avoid them.

> "I would spend hours on the internet trying to find a reason for the cancer and a treatment to make sure that my wife would be one of the 80% who made it … I couldn't let her be one of the 20%".

Our minds do not just jump back and forth like a time machine when there is an immediate threat, such as a tiger or hearing the word "cancer". They do this all the time to help us navigate through life. This is how are minds are programmed to work; it is a normal and automatic process. It helps us to feel that the world is more predictable and that we are in control.

Our minds are working in this way all the time, generating thoughts, memories, images, feelings and physical sensations. These pop up to tell us about the things we love and about the things that matter to us. When we feel threatened, they also tell us if something is wrong or that we have been pulled away from things we care about. They then 'push' us to do something about the situation as fast as possible.

"I am terrified of treatment … the thought of what I will have to go through … but I am more scared of not seeing my children grow up; so I keep going".

The overly helpful friends

It may be helpful to consider that the thoughts our minds automatically generate can be like advice from an overly helpful friend:

Imagine you are about to do something that you have never done before, such as plumbing a sink. You would like to learn the skill, but you are not sure what to do or whether it will work.

Now think about a nervous friend who is quick to point out the negatives in a situation or all the things that might go wrong. They remind you of all the times you have failed in the past. They question whether you have all the skills you need or the time to do it. When you tell them that you are now worried, they say, "that tells you that you shouldn't do it" so you don't!

Perhaps another friend would tell you "don't give up, try harder and keep at it … if you try hard enough, it will work!" They give you lots of 'helpful' advice and tell you what they would do in your situation. They tell you that you should do the same (even though they may have never done it themselves).

Then comes the friend who does not know how to do it either and so says, "Just think positive and it will all be OK".

And finally, the friend who knew someone who died from fixing his sink …

and so, you give up, exhausted!

An overly helpful friend might be pleased that they have 'saved' you from the danger of getting it wrong or making a fool of yourself. They might believe they pushed you to keep going or that they made you feel better.

What they do not realize is that in reality they may have made the situation more difficult and stopped you from doing something that could be really helpful to you.

As they think they have been helpful, they do the same again in another situation. You may be more likely to believe them as they were 'right' last time. Or maybe their voice is just too overwhelming, so you just 'give in' to what they say? Over time, we find it hard not to automatically listen to them as, underneath it all, they are a familiar voice with our best interests at heart.

You may have people in your life just like this who try to be helpful and kind in similar ways but, without realizing, could actually be stopping you from doing things that matter or leaving you feeling upset and overwhelmed.

"If one more person tells me about their aunt who had cancer but was cured by eating carrots and I should try it … I will … ".

"I am fed up with people telling me to not give up the fight … who am I fighting exactly? Me?!"

"My family are trying to be helpful, telling me what I should do but it is not their life … I know that they are trying to be kind which makes it worse".

Our overly helpful minds and the stories they tell

Just like some friends and family, our own minds can often act like an 'overly helpful friend'. One that continually tells you stories, which capture your attention with thoughts, images, opinions, ideas, judgments and feelings.

Remember, these 'stories' are trying to tell you something important about the situation you are facing and the things you care about. The stories may or may not be true. They may or may not be helpful in guiding you toward doing something that is important to you now or in your future.

Over time, you are likely to have learned to automatically pay attention to the stories your mind tells you, as if they are the truth or facts. You tune into them, listen to them and react to them. You do this without even noticing or questioning what you are doing and whether it is helpful to you. In other words, the stories 'hook' you in.

The stories may be:

- Judgment stories (about yourself, others, life, your body, your mind and what you do):

    o "It is my fault".

    o "I should be happy".

    o "The doctor got it wrong".

    o "I should be able to do what I used to do".

    o "Other people will think I'm weak".

    o "I should be able to fight this".

- About the past, such as painful memories:

    o "I can't stop picturing the room where I got my diagnosis".

    o "I should have gone to the doctor when I first felt the lump".

    o "If only I had known, I would never have …".

    o "My life has been too painful, even before this".

- About the future, such as what might happen:

    o "I won't be able to cope".

    o "I'm terrified about the treatments I might need".

- ○ "I might not live to see my children grow up".

- ○ "I am so worried about not being able to work, I won't be able to pay my rent".

- ○ "What will happen if …?"

● Why you cannot or should not do the things that matter to you:

- ○ "I miss being able to go out on my bike".

- ○ "I want to be able to look after the kids, but I am too tired".

- ○ "I'm too ill to eat so I shouldn't go to our family meal".

- ○ "I shouldn't be so close to my family; it will hurt them too much if I die".

● Rules about how life, the world or others should or should not be:

- ○ "Life should be fair".

- ○ "We are not a family who get cancer; why me?"

- ○ "People should understand".

- ○ "There must be a treatment or solution somewhere that will get rid of the cancer".

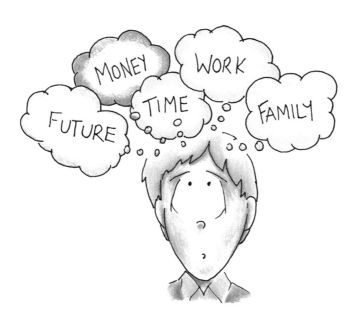

When you are coping with the impact of cancer, it can feel like you are faced with many more painful stories and 'threats' than usual. These stories can be triggered by so many things, such as something someone says, an advert on TV, going to an appointment, doing an activity you enjoy or they may even seem to pop up from nowhere.

> "When I have worries, I like to go running but now it makes it worse as all I notice is how I can't run like I used to do and then I am back thinking about 'cancer'".

"I just can't seem to clear my head, I used to pride myself on problem solving and keeping thoughts at bay … what has happened to me?"

As the 'threat' of cancer is uncertain and never goes away your mind will keep reminding you about it, even when you are doing something that you really love or enjoy. When your mind brings up the 'cancer' story, it is trying to be helpful. It is telling you to do everything you can to keep yourself safe, so you can hold on and keep connected to all the things you care about.

"I think that I am back to me when I am playing with the kids … but suddenly … boom … it hits … will I ever get to play with my grandkids? I want to be here to see them grow up so much. I have to leave the room so they don't see me upset".

"However much I try, I can never forget. I was 'cured' of my cancer over five years ago now but it takes just one person to wish me a happy birthday and I am back there … the 'what ifs' start".

However, when you are hooked into these stories, your attention is pulled away from the here and now and the things that matter to you. Your attention is dragged back into your mind and away from the world and people around you. You become stuck.

Your mind, continuing to act as an overly helpful friend, also likes to tell you more stories about the difficult thoughts and feelings themselves and what you should do when they show up.

These stories tell you that:

"You should be grateful, you are lucky!"

"You need to think of the positives".

"You should focus on what you have got".

"Just don't think about it".

"It is best not to dwell".

"You need to think it through".

"There will be a solution".

"You just have to keep going".

"You shouldn't feel like that in your situation".

"Tears are a sign of weakness".

"You need to be strong".

Ultimately, these stories that our minds tell us tend to fit into two main themes:

1. You should be able to control or get rid or your thoughts and feelings.

2. Painful thoughts and feelings are bad!

We believe these stories when they come up as they 'feel' true. We act on them as if they are factual, often without questioning it. Many people get caught up in this trap. You may find people around you share their own 'stories' with you, telling you not to worry or to look on the bright side. This can even include professionals at times.

Here are some examples:

> "My consultant has told me and my family the cancer treatment is straight-forward, and it should be, but that hasn't stopped me being worried and now I can't tell my family how I feel as the doctor told me I 'shouldn't be worried'".

> "My consultant told me that I was coping really well, but in the next appointment when she said we will need to delay the treatment I cried. She offered to refer me to counseling. I thought it was normal to cry if you heard that, so it makes me worry now that I am not coping".

So often, society and the world around us also feeds us messages that we should be 'happy' and only have 'positive' feelings. We believe that any painful or difficult thoughts or feelings that come up must mean there is a problem. Or worse, that there is something wrong with you!

> "I just feel like I am wearing a mask all the time. I can't bear to show my friends and family how much I'm struggling. If they ask me how I am I always have to pretend I'm fine. It would just upset them all too much and I don't think they would cope if they knew how I really feel. I have to keep the mask on to protect them but it's exhausting. When I'm on my own I just weep".

> "Everyone else is delighted with my scan results, but I just feel empty even though I should be happy".

The problem is not the thoughts and feelings. Painful thoughts and feelings are normal, especially when you are facing something as difficult as cancer. The problem is that you are hooked into a powerful story that tells you that you should not struggle in this way. Your overly helpful mind tells you how you 'should' think, feel and act when painful thoughts, feelings and sensations show up – that you should do everything you can to get rid of them or control them.

Getting rid of the pain or getting stuck?

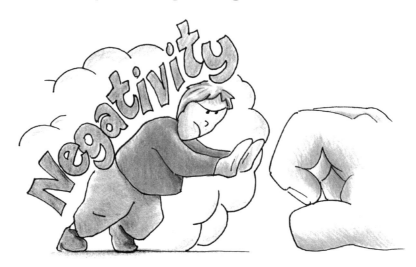

We all have many different ways of trying to get rid of difficult thoughts, feelings, memories, images and physical sensations when they show up.

Some common examples follow:

Distraction: You may try various forms of distraction (e.g. watching films back to back, surfing the internet). You might do anything that you can to keep yourself busy so you do not have to think.

"I love exercise as I don't think about my worries, but my family complain that I am always in the gym and I never see them".

"When I am worried, I clean the house, but that leaves me even more exhausted and fatigued".

Opting out: You may find yourself trying to avoid situations or people. You want to hide away from everything that reminds you of what you are facing. You may find yourself trying to block out your thoughts and feelings about it at all.

"On a bad day going out with my friends used to cheer me up, but now I struggle to see them as their lives are so different to mine. So I am staying home but I miss them so much".

"I have started avoiding my friend who keeps asking me how I am or telling me to take each day as it comes. All I can think about is that I may not be around for long!"

Thinking: You may find yourself arguing with thoughts, trying to reassure yourself; trying to find evidence that they are or are not true. You might find yourself grappling with "why?" Perhaps you try to think your way out of the problems you face, going over things in your head for hours. You might tell yourself to "pull yourself together" or criticize yourself for feeling a certain way. You think other people are to blame.

"I am fed up with people saying I should think about the positive and not to worry. Don't they think I have tried that!"

"It is going to be ok. I know it is. I am going to be one of the 50% that beats this".

Substances: You may eat, drink, take medication or even sleep to try and avoid your thoughts and feelings or difficult situations.

"When I feel sad, I eat. It makes me happy for a moment but then I worry about my weight".

"At the end of a long day, I look forward to a glass of wine … or two. It just helps me to forget".

At times you may feel overwhelmed in your struggle to manage or control the painful thoughts, feelings or sensations that come up. What you do to try and get rid of them or to control them can take up a lot of time and energy. Sometimes this may feel helpful in the short term. However, when this happens it may be keeping you stuck in the longer term. This can take you away from being the person you want to be and doing what really matters to you in life.

"I kept trying to lock the thoughts away in a box in my mind. Every time they came back, I felt like I had failed. I avoided going out and other people in case they used the word 'cancer' and it all came flooding back. I felt like the cancer had taken control".

Here is an exercise to help you to think about the strategies that you use when painful thoughts, feelings, images, memories and sensations show up, when these help you and when they may keep you stuck.

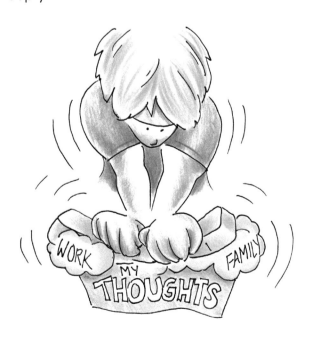

Exercise: Getting to know whether your strategies work (Russ Harris, 2019)

Write down some of the thoughts, feelings, memories, sensations or images in your mind that you would like to get rid of.

....

....

....

....

What have you done to try to get rid of these thoughts, feelings, memories, sensations and images (e.g. watch TV, gone to sleep, avoided going out, thinking 'positively', eating, planning, blaming yourself, cancelling appointments)?

....

....

....

....

How have these things helped you? How have they worked for you in the short term?

....

....

....

....

How have they worked for you in the long term?

....

....

....

....

What has this stopped you doing that you would like to be doing? What has it cost you in terms of time, energy and quality of life (e.g. talking to my friends, spending time with my children, taking my dog for a walk, feeling like I have no energy or motivation)?

....

....

....

....

Which ones have helped you to be the person you want to be? Or to do things that are important to you?

....

....

....

....

Which ones have stopped you from doing this?

....

....

....

....

You may find that some of the things you wrote down have worked well for you in the past. Some might be working right now. Some may not be working at all, but you keep trying anyway. Some might be getting in the way of you living the life you want to live.

If you are mostly using ones that are:

● Encouraging you to act in a way that you do not like,

● Moving you away from what is important to you or

● Not working at all…

…then you are likely to struggle. You may be caught up in a cycle of trying to control your thoughts and feelings or altering a situation that you cannot change. The more you struggle, the more distressing things are likely to feel. You may have discovered that this is not helping you to live a meaningful life in the long term.

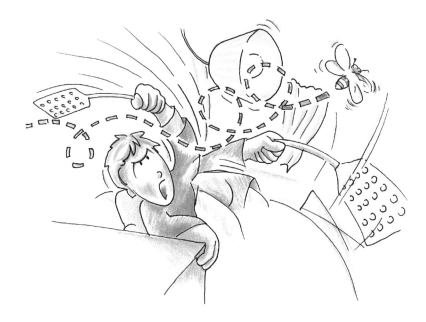

It is tough to notice that the things that you have been doing have not been working. You may be noticing some painful feelings showing up; anger, sadness, anxiety, fear … .

Your mind, as an overly helpful friend, may be giving you a hard time, criticizing you, going over times when you have been using these strategies, worrying about what you 'should' have been doing instead.

Remember, these thoughts and feelings are not the problem. The problem only occurs when you hook into a story that does not work for you. One that is 'unworkable' and holds you back rather than helping you.

Are you ready to write a new story?

In Part 2 of this book, you will learn new skills that will help you to 'drop the struggle' and sit with the painful stories, thoughts, feelings and sensations when they come up. This aims to help you to acknowledge what they are telling you and to work toward recognizing and connecting to the things you value in your life. It will also look at ways to help take the power out of the thoughts and feelings, to help you to gain a little space and perspective … to step back and notice, or 'unhook', from the stories your mind tells you. This helps you to see them for what they are … thoughts are just words and images, feelings are just sensations. From this perspective, they can't push you about so much.

Part 2 will also help you to recognize that no matter what painful stuff shows up, you are still able to do something that moves you toward a meaningful life. To do something that gives you a sense of purpose and fulfillment. There will be space within the book to help you to pause and think about what actions you can do that could add a little more meaning and fulfillment to your life. To help you to realize that although you can't control your thoughts and feelings, it is possible to take control of what you do. You can choose to do things that matter to you, even in the face of cancer and the pain it brings.

In Part 3 of the book, you will also find some practical strategies to help you to look after yourself as you navigate the impact of the cancer. These strategies are things that you may not know or have forgotten are important. These skills are also sometimes called self-care skills. They are some of the most important skills to prioritize when things get tough in life.

The following parts of this book aim to help you to learn a range of extra 'tools' to add into your toolkit, to help you to feel less threatened by your mind's normal processes and to help you recognize thoughts and feelings as just thoughts and feelings. This can help you to feel more able to choose to do what works best for you, no matter what cancer and life throws at you.

Would that work for you?

 ## KEY MESSAGES

● Being told you or someone you care about has cancer can have a massive impact on how you think and feel, as well as how much you feel able to do the things that matter the most to you.

● It is normal to experience difficult thoughts and feelings when you are affected by the impact of cancer.

● Our mind tries to keep you safe in the short term and to get rid of difficult thoughts and feelings.

● Our mind tells us stories that capture our attention, including stories that we should be happy and that we should be able to control our thoughts and feelings.

● The things we do when painful thoughts and feelings show up are helpful if they take us toward a more meaningful and valuable life. If they do not, then it can be helpful to try something different.

● This book will help you to notice when strategies are helpful for you and, if not, what else you can do to live a meaningful life.

Reference

Harris, R. (2019). *ACT Made Simple: An Easy-To-Read Primer on Acceptance and Commitment Therapy* (Second Edition). Oakland, CA: New Harbinger Publications.

2 Living a meaningful life after a diagnosis of cancer – an Acceptance and Commitment Therapy (ACT) approach to living with cancer

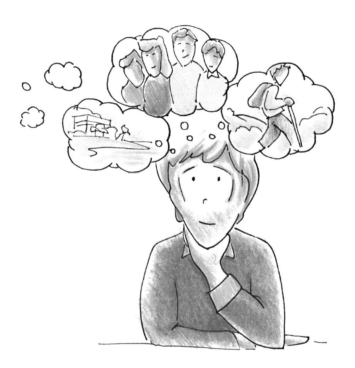

Being given a diagnosis of cancer can bring up all sorts of difficult thoughts and feelings. All the thoughts, feelings and sensations we have, whether pleasant or unpleasant, are just part of being human. We do not really have control over our thoughts and feelings, they just show up uninvited. Remember, your thoughts and feelings (even the most painful ones) are trying to tell you something important about the situation you are facing and the things you care about the most.

> "You're not going to be able to stop these thoughts and why should you? They are what make you, you".

When things are going well, our thoughts and feelings tend to be more pleasant. We are more likely to feel able to focus on doing things that we enjoy and the things that are important to us.

When things are tough and there is a big gap between how we would like life to be and how it really is – our minds and bodies are more likely to be full of painful thoughts, images, memories, feelings and sensations. We automatically get 'hooked' into them, thinking that they are relevant or important. We act as if they are true.

We then can become caught up in trying to control, get rid of or avoid these 'threats'. Our minds just keep going with this no matter what, a bit like the autopilot setting on an airplane.

This gets even trickier when something painful happens in your life, like you have been given a diagnosis of cancer. The thoughts and feelings are likely to be about the impact of cancer (such as "will my cancer come back?" and "will I die?"). No matter how hard you try, these thoughts and feelings never completely go away. Often without even noticing you find yourself struggling with these painful thoughts and feelings. You then have less time and energy to do the things in life that bring you a sense of fulfillment.

"I love chocolate when I am having a bad day; it tastes rubbish on chemo … help!"

"I just look forward to my bed when I am having a bad day, but I can't seem to stay asleep and have horrible dreams … sleep can be scary now".

"I used to talk to my friends when things were getting me down … they can listen for a bit but keep wanting to talk to me about cures or their uncle's friend's brother who 'got better'… I know they mean well but it has stopped me from talking".

"If I am having a low day and the 'black dog' is around, work used to help but I have nothing to distract me when I'm off sick".

"I seem to be able to distract myself for a moment by watching TV but then someone has a storyline relating to cancer and my mind is off; or even worse a cancer charity advert comes on … TV is no longer safe".

As you are reading this, you may notice that your mind is very busy and loud. It may be saying things like "I don't even know why I am doing some things", "sometimes I don't realize I'm doing it, so how can I stop?" or "I can't stop trying to distract myself, even though I know it is unhelpful, as I will be overwhelmed". Your mind is an expert in telling you stories that hook you in; the stories are so familiar that you may not even notice when they pop up or that they are just stories, not facts.

"Now suppose magic happens … so all these thoughts and feelings become like water off a duck's back … what would you do differently in your life?"
(Russ Harris, 2018)

To be able to live a meaningful life after a diagnosis of cancer, the first step is to learn to notice what is going on and when your mind has hooked you in. This then allows you some space to pause and 'unhook' from the story. You can then ask yourself "Is how I am responding to this story taking me toward the life I want to live? Am I doing what matters to me? Am I acting in a way that fits with how I ideally want to treat myself, others or the world?"

When life throws up distressing things like cancer, it can affect our sense of control over our lives. We forget that regardless of the thoughts, feelings, memories and sensations that show up, we are still in control of the things we do. We do not have much choice over how we think or feel (if you're unsure about this, try not to think about a green rabbit for the next few minutes) but we can choose how we act and respond.

The example below may help you to think about this:

Flying over Thunderstorms (Delduca and Johnson)

Imagine you are the pilot of an aeroplane.

After take off, you switch on the autopilot mode. This tells the plane to take over the controls and to fly itself automatically. While the autopilot is switched on, the plane keeps flying in the way it has been programmed to do.

Switching on the autopilot frees you up as the pilot to do all the other things you need to think about and do, like listening to air traffic control, making passenger announcements, monitoring the weather, ensuring everything is working as it should be, checking you are on time, eating your lunch … .

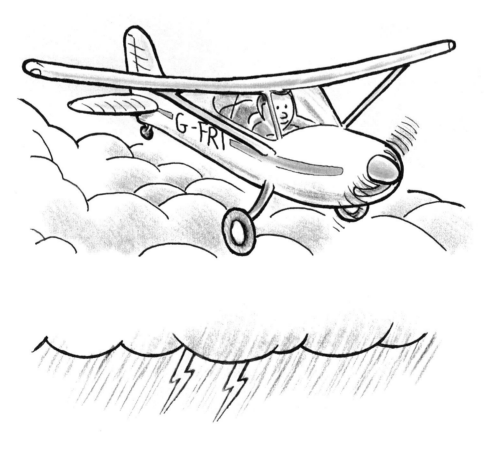

Now imagine along the route you are faced with an enormous, raging thunderstorm in front of you.

As the pilot, if you are distracted and do not notice the thunderstorm or if you choose to leave autopilot switched on the plane will keep going as pro-grammed. It will fly straight into the storm. You are likely to have a very bumpy and uncomfortable ride which feels scary, unsafe and out of your control. All you can do is hold on tight as you are buffeted about until you are out the other side. You might find yourself criticising yourself for being 'so stupid'.

Alternatively, when you first notice the thunderstorm you could take a moment and then choose to turn the autopilot off. You switch the plane off from automatic and take back manual control of the plane.

You then have more choice about what to do.

You could choose to keep flying through the thunderstorm but this time you are in charge of the plane, not the autopilot.

You could choose to avoid flying when there is a thunderstorm around, just to be on the safe side. You could find somewhere to land the plane or turn around and go back. You could try again later but you will also have cost yourself a lot in terms of time, fuel and ending up in the wrong place.

Or ...

You could choose to increase your altitude so you fly over the storm. From this height, you are able to rise above the storm clouds and even watch the lightening flashing within it. You're aware it may still be a bumpy ride, but you tell yourself you're OK. You check your compass so you know which way to head. You then decide to keep flying in the direction your compass guides you. You feel more in control of what you are doing and what hap-pens to you. You now even have some space to notice the vivid blue sky around you.

In the example above, switching on the autopilot mode is what our minds do so we can do things automatically and free up mental space. This is helpful as it enables us to use our resources more effectively. We can focus on multiple things at once (think about how it first felt to learn to ride a bike or drive a car compared to how it feels when you have been doing it for a long time). However, if we only ever keep our mind's autopilot mode switched on, we can only ever 'react' to situations we find ourselves in.

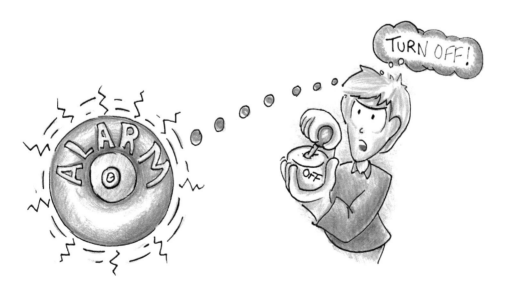

If we learn how to switch off the autopilot, we can learn to check in with what is going on around us in the here and now. We are able to notice more about the stories, situations and other things that are showing up. This gives us a little more space to consider how to respond. (Some of the techniques and exercises in this section of the book will help you to learn how to switch off the autopilot and to be more present in the here-and-now.)

Our thoughts, feelings, sensations, memories or images that show up are like the thunderstorm. We cannot control when they show up, how big they are or when they will pass. Like the weather, they all pass in their own time. When they are around and we get 'caught up' in them, it can feel uncomfortable and even frightening.

The sky in this example represents the safe space that we can learn to access inside of us from which we can notice, acknowledge and observe. From this space we can recognize the thoughts, feelings and sensations that come up and allow them to pass in their own time. This space also allows us to notice what else is around us, the small things that we can savor even in the face of great difficulties.

The compass direction we follow represents the things that matter most to us and the things that we want to build in our lives. For example, connecting to the people or things we most care about, developing the personal qualities we desire for ourselves, acting on our values and doing the things that give us a sense of purpose and fulfillment. Other people can try to guide us where to go or give us directions but ultimately nobody can tell us the right way to head, we follow our own compass.

When we take over manual control, we have more choice over what we do and where we are headed.

We can choose to do the things that our minds tell us are 'safer' or will help us to avoid any discomfort. Sometimes this can be helpful or useful to do. However, if we only ever do this, it prevents us from heading in the direction we want to go.

We can choose to do the things that take us toward our values and a meaningful life. This can sometimes feel uncomfortable but often feels meaningful and worthwhile, giving us a sense of purpose or fulfillment.

Learning to notice what shows up and how we react when we are in autopilot mode enables us to recognize when our autopilot button has been turned back on. We can then pause and choose whether to switch our autopilot off and go in to 'manual' mode instead.

This pause allows us to consider where we want to go with our lives and what actions we take. We can choose to 'respond' based on what is most helpful or workable for us (in the short and longer term), rather than 'react'.

Note: This is a metaphor that we have developed to help you to consider many of the core processes of ACT, using a real-world example. There is further information in the back of this book to explain this in more detail.

When we are able to create this awareness and space, we call this the 'choice point'.

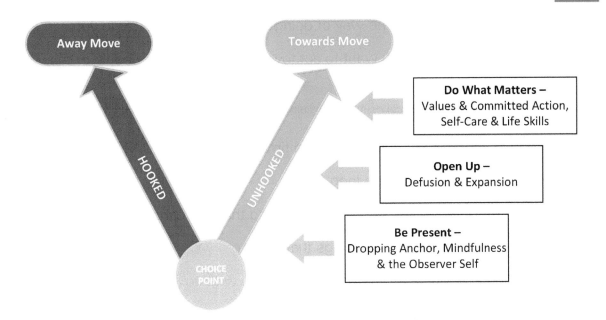

Choice Point © Russ Harris, 2017 – adapted from 'Choice Point' by Ciarrochi, Bailey & Harris (2014).

If what you do in response to your thoughts and feelings takes you toward the person that you would like to be or the future you would like to have, then we call it a 'toward move'. However, if you do something that doesn't work for you in the long term and you are acting in a way that takes you away from how you would like to be, it is an 'away move'.

What do we mean by "what you do"? As human beings we have two types of behavior: 'private' and 'public'. Private behavior, such as thinking, focusing, visualizing, mindfulness, imagining and remembering can never be seen or heard by others (despite what science fiction sometimes tells us!). Public behaviors are things you do with your arms, legs, hands and feet, facial expressions, everything you say, whisper, shout or sing; how you hold your body, breathe, move, drink and eat. If we were filming you, it would be what we see and hear you doing.

Public behavior may be something which can be seen by someone else, like eating a cake or going for a walk. Private behaviors happen in our mind, like thinking of a solution to a problem or trying not to think about something. A particular behavior may be either a toward move or an away move depending on why we are doing it. For example, if you value being with your family, watching TV and avoiding speaking with them would be an away move. If you choose to watch a TV program with your daughter that she loves (even if you don't) because you love spending the time with her, that would be a toward move.

Anything that we do to respond when we notice painful thoughts, feelings and sensations can be toward or away moves.

Actions are toward moves when:

● They fix a problem that can be fixed.

● They are used for a short period of time to help you do something that matters.

- Using them does not get in the way of doing the things that matter to you.

- You are acting in the way you want to act toward yourself, other people or the world around you.

Actions are away moves when:

- They keep us stuck or are unhelpful at the time.

- You use them too much or for a long time.

- You use them to try and control or fix something that you cannot change.

- Using them stops you doing the things that matter to you.

- You are acting in a way that is different to how you want to act toward yourself, other people or the world around you.

Remember, it is not about what you are doing. It is about why you are doing it. What matters is whether the actions move you toward a more rich and meaningful life (despite the cancer) or away from it.

"I learned that I can't control my thoughts and feelings as I'd like to, but I am in control of what I do and that is what makes a difference".

"I've learned that we're all so very different and that there's no right or wrong way of dealing with a difficult time in our lives. We each get through it in our own way and that's absolutely fine".

 KEY MESSAGES

- It is not easy to stop using strategies when they have been used for a long time and have become 'automatic'.

- The way you try and manage your thoughts and feelings can keep you 'stuck' and get in the way of you doing what you want to be doing.

- You can learn to notice what happens, what thoughts, feelings and 'stories' hook you in and how you react 'on autopilot'.

- This can give you space to think about what matters to you and whether the things you do are moving you toward or away from living a meaningful life.

So, what else can I do?

When what you are doing is taking you 'away' from the things you value most, it can help to have another set of tools in your toolkit to try instead.

The rest of this section will help you to learn ways to recognize when you have been hooked and are being pushed around by your thoughts and feelings. That is, when you are reacting on autopilot and likely to be making away moves.

It will also help you to find ways to unhook. When you unhook, you are able to acknowledge (rather than avoid) difficult thoughts and feelings when they crop up and to drop the struggle with them. This can then free up time and energy so that you can focus on doing things that matter to you, i.e. toward moves. Doing this can help you to live a meaningful life, even when things feel uncertain or tough.

ACT focuses on three main areas to help you do this:

- **Be present:** Coming back to the here and now, rather than being hooked in by thoughts about the past or future, difficult feelings, physical sensations or situations. These skills involve dropping anchor, mindfulness and becoming aware that you are different to your thoughts and feelings.

- **Opening up:** Noticing and making some space for painful thoughts and feelings; we call these skills 'Defusion' and 'Expansion' (sometimes known as acceptance).

- **Doing what matters:** Finding out what is truly important to you and the sort of person you want to be. Taking steps to do things in your life that matter, despite the cancer. This is based on your values and using skills such as 'committed action'.

These ideas and skills will be explained and explored in the rest of the book. There is a section in this part of the book which focuses on each of these ideas. We have also included some specific skills that can be helpful for when particularly painful thoughts and feelings show up, including **Urge Surfing**, and **Self-Compassion** which explores the importance of showing yourself kindness in the face of pain.

Note: within many ACT texts, you will find the word 'acceptance' sometimes refers to the process of Expansion or it can refer to letting difficult thoughts and feelings be present. From our work in cancer settings, we have found that many people struggle with the with the word 'acceptance' as they initially believe it implies that they should 'like', or 'be ok with' or 'give in' to painful experiences associated with the cancer. To avoid this confusion, we have chosen to use alternate terms in this book such as 'acknowledging' or 'being aware of' difficult thoughts and feelings and will keep to the term Expansion throughout.

Be present – Dropping Anchor, Mindfulness and the Observer Self

Dropping anchor

When we get hooked into the stories our mind tells us, it can be difficult to unhook. Sometimes we just need a moment in our day and routine to pause and remind ourselves to be present. This can be especially useful when things are feeling tough and all your painful thoughts, feelings and sensations are whirling around your mind and body, dragging you here, there and everywhere.

"When I am feeling sad, I find myself walking by the fridge and having something to eat … anything really … just to take my mind off everything".

"I feel I can only relax with friends if I have a drink in my hand … before I know it the bottle is gone".

Like a ship which is caught in a storm – rather than fighting the waves or letting your boat be battered about, it can be helpful to drop anchor until the storm passes!

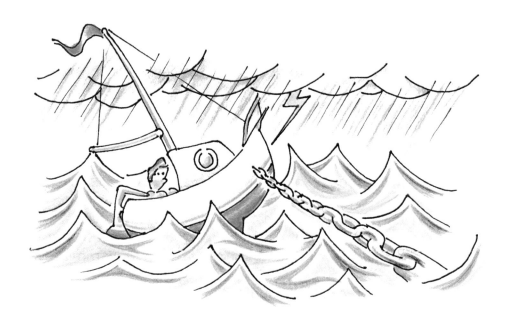

'Dropping anchor' is one of the most important skills to learn. It is a useful skill to help you to pause when difficult thoughts, feelings, emotions, memories, urges and sensations come up. It gives you a moment to switch off your autopilot and to help you to ground and steady yourself in difficult situations. It can help to:

● Disrupt rumination, obsessing and worrying.

● Focus your attention back on the present moment and the task or activity you are doing.

● Notice you are in control of your arms and legs and what you do in that moment.

● Act as a 'circuit-breaker' for impulsive, compulsive, aggressive, addictive or other problematic behaviors.

● Have space to think about whether you are engaging in life in a way that works for you right now.

● Get through short-term unpleasant situations, such as treatments or medical tests.

Exercise: So, what exactly is Dropping Anchor? (Russ Harris, 2019)

Dropping anchor involves playing around with a simple formula: ACE

A: Acknowledge your thoughts and feelings.

C: Come back into your body.

E: Engage in what you are doing.

A: Acknowledge your thoughts and feelings.

Silently and kindly acknowledge whatever is showing up inside you: thoughts, feelings, emotions, memories, sensations, urges. Take the stance of a curious scientist, observing what is going on in your inner world.

And while continuing to acknowledge your thoughts and feelings, also …

C: Come back into your body.

Come back into and connect with your physical body. Find your own way of doing this. You could try some or all of the following or find your own methods:

● Slowly pushing your feet hard into the floor.

● Slowly straightening up your back and spine; if sitting, sitting upright and forward in your chair.

● Slowly pressing your fingertips together.

● Slowly stretching your arms or neck, shrugging your shoulders.

● Slowly breathing.

You are not trying to turn away from, escape, avoid or distract yourself from what is happening in your mind and body. The aim is to remain aware of your thoughts and feelings, continue to acknowledge their presence … and at the same time come back into and connect with your body.

You are expanding your focus: becoming aware of your thoughts and feelings, while also being aware of your body while actively moving it.

And while acknowledging your thoughts and feelings, and connecting with your body, also …

E: Engage in what you are doing.

Get a sense of where you are and refocus your attention on the activity you are doing.

Find your own way of doing this.

You could try some or all of the following suggestions, or find your own methods:

● Look around the room and notice five things you can see.

● Notice three or four things you can hear or three or four elements to one sound you can hear.

● Notice what you can smell or taste or sense in your nose and mouth.

● Notice what you are doing.

● End the exercise by giving your full attention to the task or activity at hand.

Ideally, run through the ACE cycle slowly three or four times, to turn it into a two- to three-minute exercise.

It is really important not to miss out on the A of ACE. A key skill is to be able to keep acknowledging the thoughts and feelings present, especially if they are difficult or uncomfortable.

If you do not engage in A, the exercise will turn into a distraction technique – which it is not supposed to be! Distraction often pulls us away from the present moment. Acknowledging what is going on helps us to be compassionate to ourselves and to move toward a valued lifestyle.

Practice often

Remember, you can practice these kinds of exercises anytime and anyplace. It is a good idea to practice them often in less challenging situations initially, when your thoughts and feelings are less difficult, so you can build up your skill levels.

Over time, you can learn to use this in more challenging situations when your thoughts and feelings are more difficult.

If you are pushed for time, just do a 30-second version: run through the ACE cycle once or try the short version below.

If you are up for a challenge, run through the ACE cycle extremely slowly, over and over, for five to ten minutes.

There are literally hundreds of ways to modify this exercise, to accommodate your needs (e.g. physical pain) or overcome any difficulties you may have with it.

Free audio recordings

 If you wish, you can download some free audio recordings of dropping anchor exercises, varying from 1 minute to 11 minutes in length. You can listen to these and use them as a guide to help you develop this skill.

You can download or stream them from the left-hand box on this webpage: www.a ctmindfully.com.au/freestuff/free-audio/

  Exercise: Dropping Anchor (short version)

Take five to ten seconds to do the following:

1. Push your feet hard on to the floor and straighten your spine.

2. Acknowledge all the thoughts, feelings, images and sensations that are present.

3. As you do this, take a slow deep breath and notice the movement of your body.

4. Look around and notice five things you can see.

5. Listen carefully and notice five things you hear.

6. Notice five things you can feel around your body.

7. Now notice where you are and what you are doing.

If you struggle to notice five things, start with one of each. Then repeat the exercise until you can expand your awareness. The aim of the exercise is not to make you feel calm or get rid of painful thoughts and feelings. The aim is simply to give you a moment to pause when difficult things show up.

Dropping anchor can be a really helpful exercise to use by itself just to check in and to notice whether you are looking after yourself and engaging in your life in a meaningful way. You can also build on this skill with other techniques, such as mindfulness below, to help you to acknowledge what is coming up and to unhook from it.

Mindfulness

When you are given a diagnosis of cancer, your mind works hard to try to make sense of what has happened and to stop it happening again. However, because of the nature of cancer and the uncertainty that surrounds it there are usually no answers to the problems your mind is trying to solve. So, it just keeps going and going.

> "When I was told I had cancer, all I could think about was what I've done, what has happened to me in the past and worrying about my future. I couldn't understand why I have cancer. I just want to make sure it doesn't get worse or come back in the future. I can't find an answer to it".

When this happens, your mind forgets to check in with the here and now. Without checking out what is happening at that moment, you may get caught up in the stories your mind is telling you without noticing if they are helpful or not. You might believe what your mind is telling you is 'fact' and you get pulled away from taking steps toward a meaningful life. One of the skills that can be helpful when this happens is mindfulness.

Mindfulness is different from relaxation. The aim is not to feel calm. The aim is also not to make distress or difficult thoughts and feelings go away. The aim, instead, is for you to just observe and be aware of the present moment and whatever is showing up. So why is it helpful?

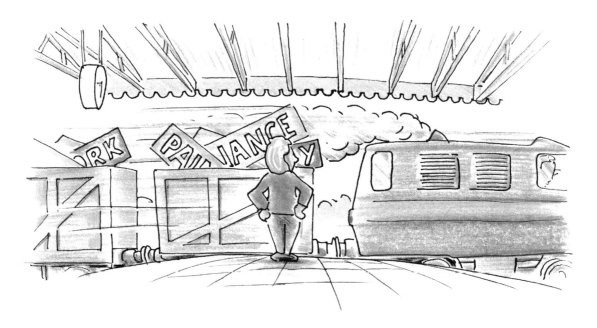

Mindfulness can help you to take a step back, notice and observe the thoughts and feelings in your mind, rather than becoming caught up in them or struggling with them. A bit like watching a train pass you by at the station rather than getting on it.

> "However much I reminded myself that I am not likely to be one of the 1% and that the scan results will be fine … the thoughts keep coming back … help!"

> "I know that I should be happy that it is gone … but has it? … that thought plagues me in the middle of the night … I do everything to talk myself out of it … remind myself of the evidence … but it comes back again … and again … and again".

Mindfulness simply means noticing what is going on in a particular way:

● On purpose.

● In the present moment.

● Non-judgmentally – allowing whatever is there to be there.

The actual skills of mindfulness might sound simple. It can take time to get used to being mindful because it is so different to our autopilot mode.

> "I used to think mindfulness was mumbo jumbo hippy stuff and not for me … then I discovered that I do it already and it isn't some mystical stuff".

"I never thought I could do it ... every time I tried my mind wouldn't empty ... and then I found out that that isn't what mindfulness is about".

"I had too much to think about with all the appointments, treatment and information I was being given. I didn't have time for it, yet another thing to do ... and then I learned that I needed to do nothing more than I was already doing ... I just had to notice things from a different angle".

It is important to remember that you will already be using mindfulness skills without even realizing. For example, when you lose track of time because you are really enjoying an activity, when you step outside the front door and notice that it is a beautiful day, when you notice the taste of your first sip of coffee.

There are some mindfulness exercises below for you to practice:

Mindful savoring

When you have lots of appointments to go to, it can feel hard to make extra time to practice mindfulness. Instead, you can add mindfulness into your daily routine, whatever you are doing. You can focus on using your senses to notice things you would not usually be aware of ... even if it is just for a moment.

For example, you could try noticing:

- The warmth of the water when you take a shower.

- The taste of your favorite snack.

- The colors of flowers in your garden.

- The sound of birds singing outside the window.

- The feel of a soft jumper against your skin.

- The feel and look of soap bubbles as you do the washing up.

When learning mindful savoring, it can be easier to start on pleasant activities. If you are experiencing difficulties with taste and smell due to being on treatment, concentrate on your other senses first such as touch, sight and sound when you practice.

Mindful walking

Walking is something most of us do at some time during the day, even if it is for a couple of minutes or a few steps. This can be a good chance to look around us and notice what we see, hear and feel. You could notice:

- The feeling of your feet as they touch the ground.

- The movement of your arms and feet as you take each step.

- The temperature of the air around you.

- The sounds of your footsteps.

- The sights around you as you walk.

As you do this, your mind may get distracted or you may notice thoughts and feelings cropping up. That is OK, once you have noticed what has come up for you, you can bring your focus back to walking.

More mindfulness exercises

Here are some more exercises that will help you to develop mindfulness skills. You can also find links to resources which have other mindfulness exercises at the end of this book.

As you try these exercises, you might notice thoughts, such as "This is weird?", "How is this going to help?", "I am hungry", "I don't like this" or "Oh, I have an itch". You may notice you are feeling calm or bored or frustrated. You may feel numb or notice 'nothing'. There is no right or wrong way of feeling for these exercises. Whatever comes up for you is OK.

Mindfulness does not stop our mind from wandering off once you are aware of the here and now. It is the process of noticing where it went and bringing it back to the here and now again and again.

  Exercise: Breathing space

1. Sit down on a chair or a cushion on the floor and sit upright with a straight back if you can. If not, you can choose to lie down.

2. Close your eyes if you feel comfortable with this.

3. Start by simply noticing your body. Notice the sensation of sitting or lying down. Notice the light pressure on your back or bottom.

4. Now, simply notice that you are breathing. Notice the sensations of breathing.

5. Observe how your chest or belly is rising on the in-breath. Notice the belly or chest falling on the out-breath.

6. Keep observing what your belly/chest is doing. Do not try to change or control it.

7. It is most likely that you will be distracted by thoughts, feelings or things going on around you. This is OK. As you notice this, gently bring your focus back to the breath.

8. Notice the sensation of the air going through the tip of your nose or through the lips.

9. Notice what the air feels like. Notice the temperature of the air.

10. If you get distracted, gently bring your focus to the breathing.

11. After two minutes, bring your attention to the body and the feeling of sitting or lying down.

12. Finally, open your eyes and become aware of your surroundings.

  Exercise: Leaves on a stream

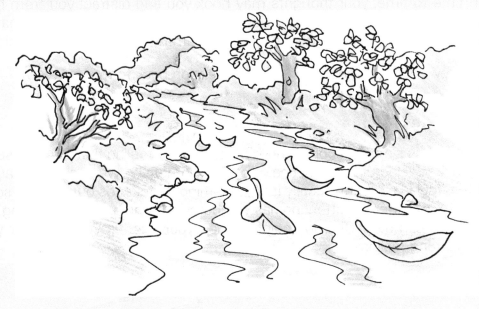

Find a quiet place and sit in a comfortable position.

1. Either close your eyes or rest them gently on a fixed spot in the room.

2. Imagine yourself sitting beside a gently flowing stream with leaves floating along the surface of the water. Imagine this picture for a few moments. (You may be able to hold the image in your mind for the exercise or you may just have little glimpses, either is OK.)

3. For the next few minutes, take each thought that enters your mind and place it on a leaf … let it float by. Do this with each thought – pleasurable, painful or neutral. Even if you have joyful or optimistic thoughts, place them on a leaf and let them float by.

4. If your thoughts momentarily stop, continue to watch the stream. Sooner or later, your thoughts will start up again. Observe your thoughts like this for a few moments.

5. Allow the stream to flow at its own pace. Do not try to speed it up and rush your thoughts along. The aim is not to try to rush the leaves along or get rid of your thoughts. Allowing them to come and go at their own pace.

6. If your mind says, "This is stupid", "I'm bored" or "I'm not doing this right", place those thoughts on leaves too and let them pass on down the stream. Keep doing this for a few moments.

7. If a leaf gets stuck, allow it to hang around until it is ready to float by. If the thought comes up again, place it on a leaf and watch it float by another time. Keep watching your thoughts for a few moments.

8. If a difficult or painful feeling arises, that is OK. Simply observe it. Say to yourself, "I notice myself having a feeling of frustration/anxiety/sadness". Place those thoughts on leaves and allow them to float along.

9. From time to time, your thoughts may hook you and distract you from being fully present in this exercise. This is normal. As soon as you realize that you have become side-tracked, gently bring your attention back to the exercise.

10. After a few more moments, bring your attention back to the room.

Having a focusing anchor

A focusing anchor is simply an object, bodily sensation or feeling that we choose to pay attention to during mindfulness practice. It can be something we can see, hear, smell, taste, touch or feel in the body. Ideally it is something that stands out enough so that it is easy to find again after our attention has wandered. Having a strong focusing anchor to come back to can be particularly helpful when your mind is very busy, or you are experiencing strong feelings.

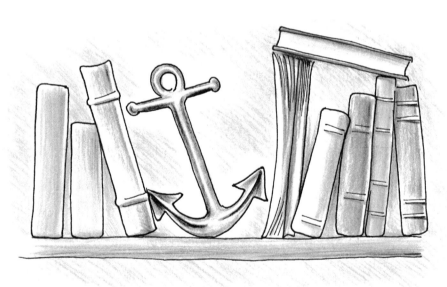

Choosing a focusing anchor

Below are some examples of what might make a helpful focusing anchor:

- **Sight:** Choose something you can see clearly and that stands out so it can easily be found again, such as tree branches/bushes/flowers blowing in the wind, cars driving past, clouds in the sky, a picture, a painting or an ornament.

- **Sound:** Try picking up on as many sounds as you can notice in your environment, such as sounds close to you, and then sounds far away. Alternatively, you can try and listen to as many elements of one sound as you can. You could try using a soundtrack of a beach/forest/river, air conditioning, birds singing, the wind, your own breathing, traffic driving past or the ticking of a clock.

- **Taste:** You can focus on the taste of one specific food or drink, or perhaps you can use various tastes and flavors with different food types in a meal. Try the taste of chewing gum/toffee/sweets or of a drink or even your toothpaste as you brush your teeth.

- **Smell:** You could use essential oils, incense, scented candles, a cup of tea/coffee, perfume or aftershave. When doing an exercise with a smell, it might be helpful to notice when you get used to the smell and at that moment move it away from your nose. At this point try noticing what aspects of the smell linger or which other smells you can notice. When the original smell has faded, bring it back up to your nose and notice it again.

- **Touch:** Notice textures, edges, temperature, firmness/softness or the weight of an object, such as a pebble or key or the wool of your jumper. You also could caress your own hand, focus on the feel of clothes or jewelry against your skin or the feeling of your hands on your chest or belly.

- **Body sensations:** This can be steady sensations such as where our feet meet the floor or body meets the chair. Or moving sensations such as walking. You could focus on the sensations of breathing.

If you are in the middle of treatment, you may find that smell and taste are difficult to use as an anchor. As senses, they can evoke difficult thoughts, feelings and physical sensations such as nausea, which may be overwhelming. As with any new skill, practice with something that is easy to anchor to and then as you gain in confidence, try other more challenging anchors.

Remember you can be mindful about pretty much anything. So just experiment with different senses and activities. Some people prefer to start with one anchor, some people like to switch between a few different anchors within one exercise.

Exercise: Focusing anchors

Write down some ideas for your chosen focusing anchors here:

....

....

....

Stepping back and observing – the Observer Self

When you are affected by cancer, it can often feel as though your thoughts and feelings take over. Lots of people feel like they just are not themselves anymore or like they have lost the 'real' them.

If you are caught up in difficult thoughts and feelings, they can feel like bullies bossing you about. It can feel like you, your thoughts and feelings are all the same thing, but …

When you have a thought, who notices it?

When you have a feeling, who feels it?

It is you who can step back and observe your thoughts and feelings. Thoughts and feelings come and go. Thoughts are just words; feelings are just sensations. You are different from your thoughts and feelings.

You are far more than just your thoughts and feelings. Thoughts and feelings are just temporary experiences. You are there watching and observing them.

This can be a tricky idea to understand. Below are some exercises to help you to explore this idea:

  Exercise: Stop and listen

Stop and silently listen to what you are saying to yourself, to the voice in your head. Once you are listening closely, consider the following points:

● Am I the thoughts that are going through my head?

● Or am I the one who is aware of these thoughts that are going through my head?

● As these thoughts are going through my head, there is a part of me that is aware that I am noticing.

● There are my thoughts and there is a part of me noticing the thoughts.

● The thoughts are changing all the time, coming and going but the part of me that is noticing the thoughts is always there.

● The thoughts are part of me, but they are not the whole of me, there is more to me than my thoughts.

The sky and weather example (Russ Harris, 2019)

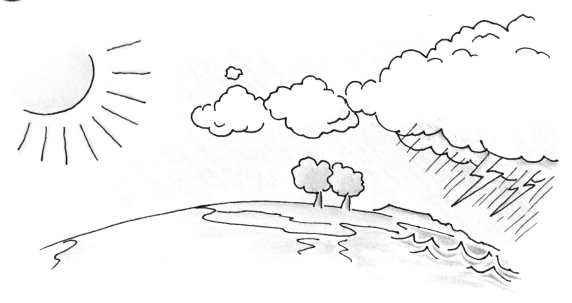

It can help to think about you and your thoughts and feelings like the sky and the weather:

- Your thoughts and feelings are continually changing, like the weather. It could be sunny one day and stormy the next.

- You are like the sky – whether you can see the sky or not, it is always there, and it always has space for the weather.

- No matter how bad the weather gets, it cannot harm the sky.

- Even if a storm is hanging around, sooner or later the weather changes.

- Similarly, your thoughts and feelings cannot hurt you. They will pass with time. You can notice and make space for these thoughts and feelings until they pass.

- You are the same 'you' that has always been there since you were small.

Noticing that you are different from your thoughts and feelings and then practicing mindfully observing them can help you to step back and unhook from them. Difficult thoughts and feelings come and go on their own. Sometimes they hang around, sometimes they go quite quickly. Like the clouds in the sky, they will all eventually pass – without you needing to put time or effort into controlling them or pushing them away.

"Being able to see that your thoughts are only thoughts and feelings are only feelings and are not you is helpful".

"This thing of 'you are not your mind'; that had never connected with me, I always felt this thing constantly pushing me, criticizing me, I thought you just had to put up with it, it was part of life … so watching my thoughts and thinking about what is it that I am actually doing now, what's important now, that was really helpful".

Once you are able to drop anchor and acknowledge your thoughts and feelings without them hooking you in, it can give you the chance to choose what you want to do in response to them; to notice whether your actions are taking you toward or away from the person you would like to be and the life you would like to live.

 KEY MESSAGES

- Most of the time our mind automatically thinks about the past or worries about the future.

- Dropping anchor and mindfulness skills can help you to stay in the here and now; to be present and to allow thoughts and feelings come and go in their own time.

- Thoughts and feelings can come and go without you putting time and effort into trying to get rid of them.

- There are exercises to help you to develop mindful awareness and to notice that you are different from your thoughts and feelings.

Open up – Defusion and Expansion techniques

This section is about opening up, which means making space for difficult thoughts and feelings. It will look at three techniques:

1. **Defusion:** A way to drop the struggle with difficult thoughts.

2. **Expansion:** A way to make space for difficult thoughts and feelings.

3. **Urge Surfing:** Learning to 'ride the wave' of the most painful feelings or to ride the urge to avoid difficult thoughts, feelings and sensations.

When particularly painful, threatening or distressing thoughts, feelings, images or emotions have shown up and you have dropped anchor, it can be really difficult not to be hooked straight back and then react to them automatically. For example:

"My cancer has come back".

"My scan results are going to show it's worse".

"I'm not going to be able to cope".

"I'm going to die".

At times like these, you can keep dropping anchor and then use Defusion and Expansion strategies to engage with them in a different way.

"Your mind sort of bullies you into a certain direction and you can decide to take a different direction if you want to".

Before we introduce Defusion and Expansion, here is an exercise that may help you to understand more about the effect of the difficult thoughts that go around in your head and the painful feelings that show up.

  Exercise: Passengers on the bus – getting to know your thoughts and feelings

Imagine the following:

- You are a bus driver. You start off on the bus route with a few passengers. You make regular stops along the route. Passengers get on and off at each stop. Most of the passengers sit and chat quietly and calmly. But a few are noisy, rude and troublesome.

- The troublesome passengers shout things like

   o "Hurry up! Don't keep stopping!"

   o "Don't go there, turn here instead".

   o "The bus will never get down there, turn around".

   o "Pull over and stop the bus".

   o "You are a useless driver".

- Some passengers say nice things:

   o "Don't listen to them, you are a good driver".

   o "Isn't the view lovely".

- Other passengers say neutral things:

   o "My stop is coming up next".

   o "I'm going shopping in town today".

- The troublesome passengers are like the difficult thoughts you might have, such as

   o "The cancer is coming back".

   o "Treatment isn't working".

   o "I am a burden to others".

   o "I am not able to care for others as well as I would like to".

   o "I have lost most of what is important to me".

- As the bus journey progresses, you notice you are feeling more and more irritated with the noisy passengers. You start to think about what you can do about them.

- You could stop the bus and order them to get off, but they might simply refuse to do so or get louder and more disruptive. The longer you stop to argue with them, the longer it holds up your bus journey.

- You could do what they tell you and drive faster or not stop at all at the bus stops, but this won't help you to be the safe, helpful and responsible bus driver you want to be.

- You could try and ignore the noisy passengers and only listen to the 'positive' ones, but you might miss a turning or a bump in the road as you are looking at the view.

- Instead, you could remind yourself that they are all just passengers that come and go along the route; they are not driving the bus. You are driving the bus and can choose which route to go (despite what the passengers say) and what sort of driver you want to be.

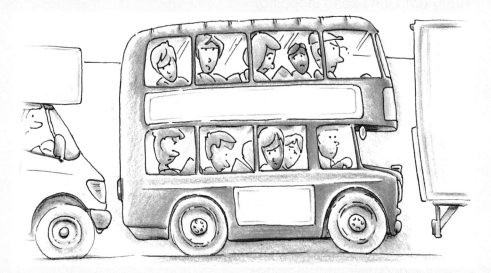

 ### Exercise: Who are the passengers on your bus?

Imagine you are the bus driver in the example above. Make a list of the passengers you often have on your bus. What do they say to you? How do they make you feel?

....

....

....

....

....

"Before, I never got to where I wanted to go; I was always getting distracted by my passengers who were bossing me about; 'it will come back', 'why are you wasting your time' … when I took control of the steering wheel and concentrated on the road ahead … I kept going even with my difficult passengers".

"Being in control and driving that bus yourself, it just builds your confidence again".

Defusion – changing your relationship with difficult thoughts

Like the passengers on the bus, our minds are incredibly good at making us pay attention to the stories they tell us. Our minds tell us that these stories and thoughts are important, especially when they are about the impact of the cancer and survival. We get hooked into these thoughts and react to them in the same way we would fight or run away from the hungry tiger. Even if we try to control the thoughts, they may go away for a time but more often than not they come back.

 For example, try the following exercise:

- Think about your favorite food. Imagine the taste of it, the smell, where you would be eating it, who you are with etc.

- Now, for the next minute, try not to think about that favorite food. If thoughts about that food come up, do whatever you can to make them go away.

- Did thoughts about your favorite food come up? What strategies did you use to make these thoughts go away? How much effort did it take you?

- Now, for the next minute, allow you mind to run free. If you think about your favorite food, that is OK. If your mind wanders elsewhere, that is OK too.

- Did thoughts about your favorite food come up this time? Did you think about your favorite food more, less or the same as the first time? How much effort did it take you compared to the first time?

Often in this exercise people find that they think about their favorite food more when they are trying to control their thoughts and make them go away.

This effect can be even stronger when you are trying to get rid of thoughts that are worrying, such as your mind's stories about cancer, treatment, uncertainty about your future and worries about dying.

If you become hooked in when these thoughts come up, you start to believe all these stories are true. You might find you give the stories lots of attention. You might feel stuck or 'fused' with the thoughts. This can feel like a big struggle.

As we learned in the previous section, thoughts and feelings can come and go in their own time without us needing to work hard to get rid of them. However, it can feel difficult to sit with this, as they feel so threatening and scary.

You may have been told by other people, "Don't worry, it'll all be OK", "You'll be fine" or "Just think positively". This might have made you try even harder to get rid of your worries. You might find yourself thinking that you have failed when you cannot do this.

So, what can you do instead?

Learning to 'defuse' from your thoughts can help you to see them for what they really are ... just a series of words or pictures in your mind.

It is not important whether the thoughts are true or untrue. What is important is whether they help you to live a meaningful and fulfilling life at that moment.

> "The thought that 'I want to go to sleep' isn't helpful when I need to get to an appointment and haven't got time to have a nap".

> "I can't stop thinking about not being here anymore; I know I haven't got as much time as I want and I feel such grief. I don't want to think about it, but it makes me ask myself whether I'm living the life I want now".

  ### Exercise: Defusion "I have the thought that ..." (Russ Harris, 2019)

Step 1

- Pick a thought that comes up for you that you struggle with. For example, "I'm a burden to my family".

- Write the thought down on a piece of paper.

- Read the thought out loud slowly to yourself over and over for 30 seconds. Get caught up in it, believe it as much as you can.

- Notice what else comes up for you ... any other thoughts, feelings, sensations, memories and images?

Step 2

● Just above your original thought, write down "I am having the thought that ...". Keep the original thought the same (e.g. "I am having the thought that I'm a burden to my family").

● Read the whole sentence out loud slowly to yourself over and over for 30 seconds.

● Notice what else comes up for you ... any other thoughts, feelings, sensations, memories and images?

Step 3

● Now, just above your thought, write down "I notice that ..." Keep the original thought the same (e.g. "I notice that I am having the thought that I'm a burden to my family").

● Read the whole sentence out loud slowly to yourself over and over for 30 seconds.

● Notice what else comes up for you ... any other thoughts, feelings, sensations and memories?

Step 4

● Turn the piece of paper over and give the thought a title, like the name of a story book (e.g. "The Burden Story").

● Next time the story comes up for you, notice it and name it (e.g. "Aha, there is "The Burden Story" again!").

You may have noticed that going through the steps above gave you some space from the thought or made the thought seem less powerful. This can happen even though you said the same words each time. This is Defusion.

The aim of Defusion is not to get rid of or change the thought. Instead, it is noticing the thought and allowing the thought to be there. It can be like taking a step back from the story. (Note: if this exercise brought up painful or difficult feelings, it might help to try the dropping anchor exercise or the Expansion exercise in the next section.)

If you can defuse from the thoughts, you can then choose whether to pay attention to the thought. If it is telling you something important, then you can choose to act on it. Or you can choose to drop the struggle and let it pass by.

> "Saying the thought 'I have cancer' was terrifying ... I didn't want to do it ... it felt as if it would become overwhelming ... doing the exercise shocked me ... it didn't change the fact that I have cancer ... but I suddenly felt a space and that I was still me".

As in the quote above, the same can happen for words that make you feel worried or upset when you hear them, even if they did not cause you any distress before. For example, words like scan, hospital, results, journey, battle, fight and brave. Defusion can help you with these words too. Try the exercises below:

 ### Exercise: Other Defusion exercises

- Repetition is another way to help take the 'sting' out of a troublesome or hurtful thought.

- Pick a neutral word, such as "lemon" and say it out loud.

- What thoughts, images, smells, tastes or memories come up for you?

- Now repeat the word out loud over and over as fast as possible for 30 seconds (this works better if you say it aloud rather than in your mind).

- What comes up now? Does it become just sounds or lose its meaning?

- Now try this with a word or phrase that you struggle with, such as "cancer", "I can't bear this anymore", "I'm worthless" or "I'm going to die".

Most people find repeating a word or phrase turns the volume down and makes it less powerful and less likely to hook them in.

Other ways of defusing you can try include:

- Sing the thought along to a tune like "Happy Birthday", in your normal voice, then change the pitch to very high and then very low.

- Imagine the thought being spoken by a cartoon character, a sports commentator or in different accents from across the world.

- Imagine the thoughts written on a computer screen – what happens if you change the size, color or font of the thought?

- Simply watch your thoughts and allow them to come and go in their own time like leaves floating by on a stream, passing cars, drifting clouds, suitcases on a conveyor belt, bubbles rising or trains pulling out of a station.

- Say thanks to your mind when you notice unhelpful or painful thoughts. It is really important to use a kind tone of voice, rather than a sarcastic or critical tone.

When doing these exercises, you may notice that you haven't been wondering whether the thought is true or false or trying to get rid of it or turn it into a 'positive' thought.

This means that you have defused from it and are starting to see it for what it is, just words!

"I tried so hard not to say the word 'cancer'; instead, we called it the 'C word' but it would still take me straight to all those feelings and thoughts. Doing the exercise taught me that it is just a word and not scary in itself ... I felt free from hiding from the word. I still didn't like it, but I stopped needing to avoid it".

Defusing from a thought gives you space to ask yourself if the thought is helpful to you or not in that moment.

Ask yourself the following questions:

- Is this thought in any way useful or helpful?

- Is this a dusty old story? Have I heard this one before?

- What would I get for believing in this story?

- Could this be helpful? Or is my mind just babbling on?

- Does this thought help me to do something important to me?

- If I follow what this thought is telling me, does it help me to do something meaningful? Or do I end up struggling with it?

- Does this thought help me to be who I want to be?

By doing this you can then choose whether to act on this thought or not.

"Rather than listening to those things [critical thoughts] ... you need to not struggle with them, let them flow over you".

"I take things a bit at a time now ... or look at things in a different way ... so I'm feeling more like me again".

 KEY MESSAGES

- It is normal to notice thoughts that tell you unhelpful or upsetting stories.

- You may find you become hooked or caught up in these stories.

- If this happens, you can try Defusion strategies to drop the struggle with the thoughts.

- You can then ask yourself if these thoughts are helpful or not for guiding you toward a fulfilling life.

Expansion – allowing difficult feelings to be there

Expansion (also known as acceptance) is a way to open up and make room for feelings and sensations, including the ones you would rather not have or usually struggle with.

Acceptance of feelings does not mean liking or wanting the feelings. It is also not about 'giving in' to feelings or 'putting up' with them. It is instead about allowing all feelings to be present when they come up, whether they feel nice or not, and making space for them to be there.

Just like our thoughts, it can be very hard to control how we feel.

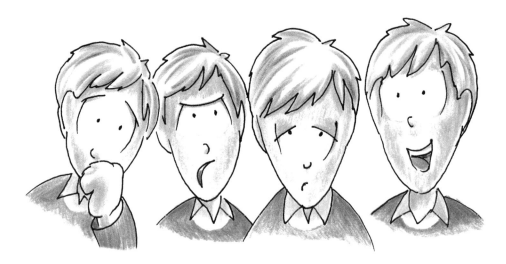

 Exercise: Can you really control your feelings?

- Imagine that the next person to walk through the door is a world-famous cancer specialist.

- This person will give you the cure for your cancer and make sure it will never come back again.

- There is one condition, they will only give you the cure if you can genuinely make yourself fall head over heels in love with them the moment they walk through the door.

- Could you do it?

You might find yourself saying "Yes, I would try!" There would be a very good reason to try hard to feel this way if it could help you to be certain that the cancer would go away forever. However, ask yourself again could you genuinely make yourself fall truly in love?

Even if you really wanted the cure, it would be very difficult to make yourself feel a particular way.

We like to think that we can control our feelings. You may have been told "You're lucky you've got such as good team treating you", "Great news, you've finished treatment, you should feel happy!" or "Cheer up, there are people who have it worse". However, most people who have been affected by cancer just do not feel like this.

> "I have been discharged as I am 'cancer free', my family and friends want to throw a party, but I feel terrified as my safety net is gone, why don't I feel happy?"

> "People have said 'at least you're here to tell the tale' or 'you're one of the lucky ones'. Well yes that's true, but you don't feel very lucky after what you've been through and then there's the constant fear of it coming back. I feel guilty for not being grateful".

Like with thoughts, you might find it hard to notice that you do not feel happy, relieved or 'positive' when you or other people expect you to feel this way. This is because your mind just wants you to survive – it keeps telling you stories about dangers and threats that might come up in the future. This might bring up painful feelings of fear, uncertainty or sadness.

These feelings often get called 'negative' feelings. We often do not like them. They can feel overwhelming or another thing to cope with on top of all the treatment and side effects that you may be managing.

However, these feelings are not 'negative' – they tell you that there are things in life you really care about. The exercise below may help you to see how important feelings are, even the most difficult ones.

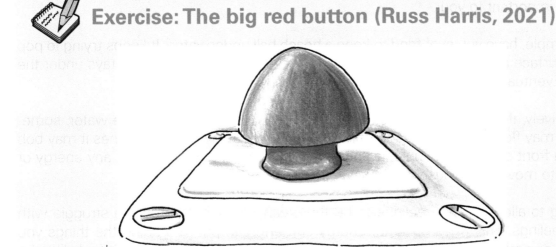

Exercise: The big red button (Russ Harris, 2021)

- You are given a big red button.

- If you press the button, then all the feelings you don't like or want, like pain, sadness, fear, frustration and anger, will disappear.

- There is only one side effect – if you press the button, you won't care about anyone or anything anymore.

- Would you press the button?

Most people would hesitate or choose not to press the button. However, some people would still choose to press it if they are in a crisis or they just feel they cannot find a way to carry on right now. If you feel like this, it is important to seek additional help. There are many support services that can help you. You can find details about some of these services in the resources section at the back of this book.

Remember, all the feelings we have, whether pleasant or unpleasant, are just part of being human! They all tell us something important about what we value and the things that matter most to us in life.

When the gap between what you want and what you have got is small, you may notice more pleasant feelings. When something has happened in your life that feels like a slap in the face or a painful blow, like cancer, this often means the gap is bigger and you may feel more unpleasant feelings.

> "I am so sad that I cannot look after my grandchildren after school but if I didn't feel sad it would mean that they don't matter to me".

> "I could have walked round with blinkers on if I wanted but I had to accept that I'd had cancer and I needed to learn to deal with the aftermath of it".

When painful feelings come up, we often automatically try to bury the feelings, to push them away, ignore them or distract ourselves from them. It can give temporary relief from difficult feelings. However, this does not make the feelings go away. Often the feelings will come back, and you will just have to put more and more energy and effort into pushing them away. What is more, all these approaches to getting rid of 'bad' feelings take up time and energy. They stop you putting this time and energy into things that are important to you.

For example, have you ever tried to keep a beach ball underwater? It keeps trying to pop to the surface and you must try harder and harder to make sure that it stays under the water. Eventually, you get tired and it flies into the air.

Alternatively, if you allowed the beach ball to float on the surface of the water, sometimes it may float near to you, sometimes it may float away and sometimes it may bob about in front of you for a while. It does this without you needing to put any energy or effort into moving it or pushing it away.

Learning to allow all your feelings to be there can help you to drop the struggle with these feelings. This frees up time, energy and effort to put into doing the things you want to do and being the type of person you want to be … even when it feels like the cancer is getting in the way.

The more you can open up and give feelings room to move, the easier it is for your feelings to come and go without effort and without them holding you back or pulling you away from where you want to be.

You may also start to learn more about your feelings. For example, where in your body you feel worry or sadness and any other sensations, feelings or thoughts that come along too.

You may find this helps you to feel that you know yourself a bit better and to learn that you can sit with difficult emotions and thoughts when they arise.

Remember that making space for difficult feelings does not come naturally to us. From an early age, we are all programmed to try to 'fix' things that bother us. So, we need to learn this skill. Here are some exercises that will help you to practice sitting with difficult feelings, so the process becomes more familiar.

  Exercise: Expansion (Russ Harris, 2019)

When you notice a difficult feeling coming up, try the following steps:

- Quickly scan your body from head to toe. Observe the emotions and sensations that are coming up for you, as if you are noticing them for the very first time. What can you feel? Where is the feeling in your body? Where is it most intense? Name the emotion you feel.

- Take a slow and deep breath. Imagine your breath flowing into and around the feeling.

- See if you can open up a little around the feeling, make some room for the feeling to be there. See if you can give it some space.

- You do not need to like, want or approve of the feeling. Just see if you can allow it to be there.

- Imagine the feeling is an object, what shape does it have, what color and texture? Does it change shape? Is it moving or is it still?

- Notice that you are bigger than this object – no matter how big it gets it can never get bigger than you.

- Remind yourself that this feeling is normal; it is part of being human and it tells you about the things that matter to you and that you care about.

- Treat yourself with kindness and compassion – place a hand gently over the area you feel the feeling most strongly and notice the warmth flowing into your body. Hold it gently.

- Begin to expand your focus of awareness. Notice the other sensations in your body, notice the sights and sounds around you, move your body around a little and take a stretch – in this moment there is you, this feeling, your body, other sensations and feelings, a room, other people and a world around you.

You can also use this exercise for feelings and body sensations that crop up for example, when you are in pain or fatigued.

When feelings show up you may find it helpful to ask yourself if:

● You can hold this feeling gently?

● You can create space for this feeling?

● You can treat this feeling like a guest?

● You can allow this feeling to come and go freely without a struggle?

● You are willing to have that feeling to do what matters?

Some people find it helpful to silently say to themselves:

● "I don't like this feeling, but I have room for it".

● "It's unpleasant, but I can allow it".

> "When doing the Expansion exercise, I suddenly realized that the feelings cannot get bigger than me; I am not going to explode, and it will be OK. Suddenly, I feel hope".

 ## KEY MESSAGES

● Trying to fight with or get rid of feelings can leave you struggling and can make you feel frustrated and distressed too.

● In the same way as you did with thoughts, you can allow feelings to be there.

● Learning to make space for feelings can free up time and energy to focus on being true to yourself and living the life you want to live.

Urge Surfing

When you are coping with the impact of cancer, you are likely at times to experience some very strong and painful feelings. Sometimes an unpleasant feeling can feel overwhelming. You might feel strong sensations in your body too. You may have a powerful urge to fight or get rid of these feelings and sensations. You might feel that your autopilot is stuck on, pushing you to keep fighting and experiencing the pain.

Hooking into the urge to get rid of a feeling can quickly pull you away from being the person you want to be. Or doing things that matter to you.

It can help to remember that an urge can be like a wave. It builds up, peaks and then breaks. Like thoughts and feelings, urges pass in their own time. We can learn to surf the urge wave!

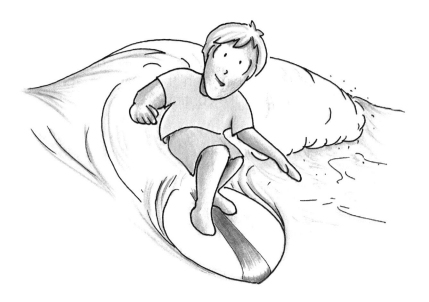

Imagine you have had a scan and you are waiting for the results. The uncertainty about the results is making you feel very worried. You have an urge to keep calling your nurse to find out if the results are in. You cannot always get through and when you do, the nurse does not have any more information to give you. The nurse tells you he will call you when he has the information. Continuing to call is not getting you the answer you need. You want to go to see your family, but you are worried you might miss the nurse calling back. The worry and urge to call is rising again. Below is an exercise that might help in this kind of situation.

  ### Exercise: Surfing an urge

- Step 1: noticing the unpleasant sensation or urge. Notice the different elements within it. Where do you feel the urge or sensations in your body? It could be helpful to name the sensations, feelings or urges. For example, "I am feeling anxious" or "I'm having the urge to pick up the phone". Rate how strong it is out of 10.

- Step 2: Once you have noticed the urge bring your attention on your chosen focusing anchor. (See the exercise above in the second section of Part 2.)

- Step 3: Mindfully focus on your anchor for a while.

- Step 4: Check in with the feeling/urge again. Has it strengthened or lessened at all? Rate it out of 10 again.

- Step 5: Continue Steps 1–4 until the wave of the urge has passed.

- Step 6: If the urge wave begins to peak again, begin again at Step 1.

- Step 7: As time passes, you may begin to notice that even when the urge is present you can still move your arms and legs.

- Step 8: Ask yourself, what is the most helpful/important thing for me to do right now?

Once you have done this, congratulate yourself for surfing the urge. It can be hard to learn at first but, with time, your confidence that you can sit with the urge will grow. Learning to surf an urge can help you to have space to choose to do something that matters – like going out to see your family in the example above, rather than doing something that is keeping you stuck – like continuing to call.

After using Defusion, Expansion and particularly, Urge Surfing, you may need to look after yourself for a while! Below is one way to do this. It is called 'self-compassion'.

Self-compassion – being kind to yourself

Facing uncertainty or other difficult thoughts and feelings can be very painful. You might find yourself becoming caught up with self-critical thoughts, such as "I'm a burden", "I'm not good enough", "I should be OK for my family's sake" or other stories your mind tells you about how you should feel.

Learning to sit with these feelings or surf urges that arise can feel tough. It is important to take care of yourself when these thoughts and feelings arise, especially during what can be a very stressful time in your life.

You may look to other people to help you and care for you at this time. It can be especially tough if people around you struggle to understand how you feel or to give you the care you need. You may understandably feel sad, let down, resentful or angry.

At these times, the only person who you can completely rely on to know exactly what you need and to give you this understanding and kindness is … you. This can be a strange idea to consider at first. To help explain this further, take a moment to think about the following quote:

> "Holding on to anger is like grasping a hot coal with the intent of throwing it at someone else. You are the one who is getting burned".
> *(Buddhaghosa;* Visuddhimagga *IX, 23)*

If we hold on 'tightly' to self-critical thoughts, resentment or anger, we can end up hurting more. We may become upset about the fact we feel anger or resentment, then frustrated that we feel upset, then even more critical stories of ourselves are likely to arise and then we feel hopeless and out of control.

It can be hard to recognize when we are holding the 'hot coals' of painful thoughts and feelings tightly. Learning to become aware of when this is happening can help you to recognize when you could drop anchor or use any of the skills we have explored above.

By doing this, it can help you to learn to:

● Acknowledge and recognize the core pain (burning sensation) that is showing up for you in that moment.

● Notice what important values that this pain may be telling you about.

● Give yourself permission to forgive yourself for what has gone before.

● Show yourself compassion.

In the same way you may offer care to someone else who is struggling, you could choose to show kindness and understanding to all of yourself, including all the distressing thoughts and pain that you are experiencing in these moments.

Ask yourself:

- Can I hold myself, and all the pain and distress I am experiencing, with kindness, compassion and forgiveness?

This can be as simple as acknowledging to yourself:

"This really hurts, this is hard" or "I know this hurts but I can do this".

Other people may struggle to understand your feelings and needs as they could still be caught up in their own stories about trying to get rid of your pain. Learning to show yourself compassion can also help you to give yourself permission to share your feelings with others to help them to understand, or to simply let them out with someone you trust. It could also help you to give yourself permission to ask for or accept help at times when you need it.

Below is a self-compassion exercise for you to try:

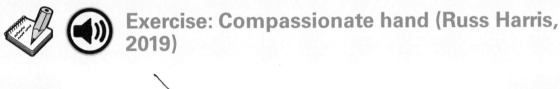

Exercise: Compassionate hand (Russ Harris, 2019)

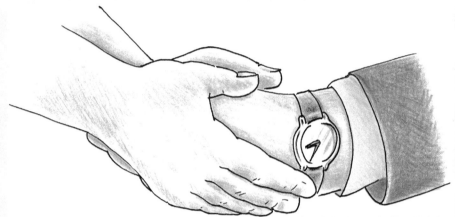

1. Sit in a comfortable position, straighten your back, drop your shoulders and press your feet gently into the floor.

2. Take a moment to notice the pain you are experiencing now, and any other thoughts and feelings that come with it.

3. Pick one of your hands and imagine it is the hand of someone very kind and caring. Place this hand on the part of your body where you feel the feeling (or numbness) most strongly. Allow your hand to rest gently on this area and feel the warmth flow from your palm into your body.

4. Imagine your body softening around the difficult feeling, making space for it to be there. Hold the difficult feeling gently, with caring and warmth. As if you are reaching out to someone you care about, let kindness flow from your fingers into your body.

5. Now place one of your hands on your chest and the other on your stomach. Let them rest there and hold yourself kindly. Take as long as you wish to sit like this, caring for yourself; giving yourself comfort and support.

KEY MESSAGES

- When difficult thoughts and feelings come up, you can use techniques like dropping anchor, mindfulness, Defusion, Expansion, Urge Surfing and self-compassion.

- Struggling to get rid of thoughts and feelings can unintentionally cost you a lot in terms of time, energy and effort. This can take you away from living a meaningful life in the face of cancer.

- Making space for difficult thoughts and feelings to be present can help you to acknowledge what is coming up for you and what matters to you.

- It can help you to press 'pause' and notice what you can change, what you can influence and what is out of your control.

- It is important to give yourself permission to be kind and compassionate to yourself when you are struggling and to acknowledge that things are hard.

- Once you have looked after yourself, you can use the extra time and energy to do something that matters to you; a toward move.

Do what matters – Values and Committed Action

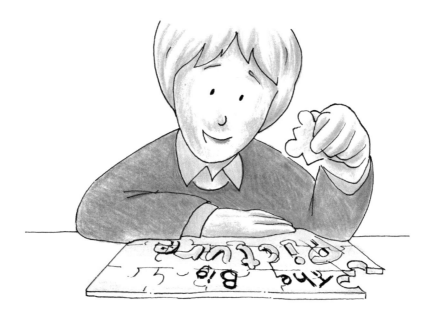

It can sometimes be difficult to think about why you might allow painful thoughts and feelings or uncertainty to be there. As you practice the ways of doing this outlined in the Defusion, Expansion and Urge Surfing sections above, you might notice your mind asking, "what is the point?"

Noticing difficult thoughts and feelings can help you to reconnect with the things that you care about most when it feels like the impact of the cancer has got in the way of this. Dropping the struggle with these thoughts and feelings can free up a little time and energy.

Remember, even though you cannot control your thoughts and feelings, you still have control over what you do. Even when the strongest urge, feeling, thought or sensation arises, you can still move your arms and legs to do something that matters.

You can invest the time, energy and effort into doing something that gives you a greater sense of purpose, meaning or fulfillment in your life, even in the face of pain!

> "I was overwhelmed when I noticed that I don't actually explode with anger or anxiety … the feelings can't get bigger than my body even when they are so painful … in a strange way it has given me a sense of control".

> "Cancer was and is the hardest thing that I have ever faced in my life and it keeps hitting me even though I am two years after treatment … despite this I have learned that I can still be me".

You may find you need to think about what to do with the time and energy you save. You might want to make this time count, to do things that matter to you. The next section will help you to find out what is important to you so that you can decide which toward moves you want to invest your time and energy in.

Values

You may well have noticed that certain things you have done in your life have felt very meaningful and important to you. These are likely to be things which have been in line with your values. Values are things like being generous, compassionate, kind, caring, adventurous, honest, reliable, dependable, curious, considerate of other people's feelings, etc.

Connecting to our values may feel enjoyable. However, sometimes you may have connected to your values because it is important to you even though it feels painful to do so.

> "I just can't bear the treatment … it is terrifying, but I want to be with my family … but I want to be there to love them and treatment is my best chance to do it".

> "I find it so hard to listen to my friends talking about 'small' stuff. I want to avoid them or shout at them … 'I have got cancer; your problems are nothing' … but then I wouldn't be the caring friend that I want to be".

It can help to think about what your values are because when life gets rough, it can be easy to lose sight of them.

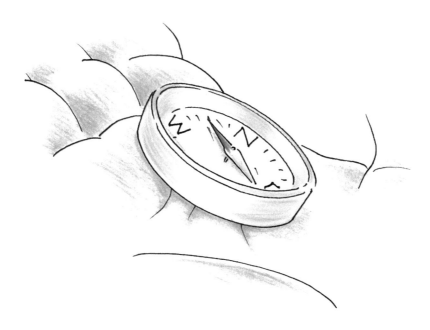

Think of your values as a compass and you as the captain of a ship or an airplane. The compass helps to guide your journey, even when it is dark and a storm is raging. Values help to keep you on course to head in the direction you want your life to go, even when painful thoughts, feelings and situations show up.

"Working out our values and things was useful because it does make you evaluate what your life was like before, what was important. It makes you think how you've come through, what is important now and how you can move forward".

"For me, I've been thinking how I have always loved being outside and in nature. That's where I get a lot of my enjoyment. That hasn't changed. In fact, maybe I have more time for that now".

Let's illustrate this with an example of how values can affect our approach to cancer. You will notice it is not entirely straightforward since different values can pull you in different directions!

You might value treating your partner, children or friends in certain ways – being caring, protective, supportive, patient or understanding. You might also value honesty and openness. Your overly helpful mind might alert you strongly to avoid telling your family and children about the cancer to protect them from worry. However, this involves keeping secrets and lots of effort to appear 'OK' on the outside. It is also hard to go against your value of being open and honest. And anyway, despite all your efforts to hide it, your family will probably have still noticed something is wrong or different.

It can be very painful to tell your family about the cancer, but in the long run it can help you all to feel closer. You can help your children and family to understand the cancer, the changes you face and support them with their worries. In turn, they can offer you support which is helpful to you as they know more about what you need.

> "I was so afraid to tell my children about the cancer, but it was exhausting keeping secrets. It felt like there was a wall in between us and no matter how hard I tried to hide it they knew something was wrong … in the end, as hard as it was to tell them, we now feel closer again and we talk openly together about our worries".

What are values?

There are no 'right' or 'wrong' things to value (notice when your mind tells you stories that there are values that you 'should' or 'should not' hold and see if you can defuse from these thoughts). Values are personal choice and just the things that are important to you.

Think about the following questions to help you think about what you value:

- Like a compass – which direction do you want your life to head in, even when the road gets bumpy?

- Desired qualities – what sort of person do you want to be, despite the cancer? How do you want to behave toward yourself, others and the world?

- Different from rules and goals – deep down, what matters to you? What do you care about? What do you want to stand for?

- What gives you a sense of fulfillment, purpose and meaning in life?

At its simplest, values are often the things we care about, connect to or something we find it fulfilling to contribute to. In the face of life's difficulties, or painful thoughts and feelings, your values can keep you going and guide you in your choice about how to act in a way that is meaningful to you. Your values can be especially helpful to consider when you notice you have been hooked by your thoughts and feelings and these are pushing you away from the things that matter. Instead you are caught up in avoiding, or trying to cut off or escape from something.

> "When I recognized that I could still be creative even though I couldn't paint anymore, I felt a huge sense of release".

> "I can still feel a sense of achievement, I can't run marathons, but I have set myself a different goal – I am learning Spanish … Hola!"

> "Since I have not been able to look after my grandchildren after school, I have felt such a loss … I realized that I can still care for them, I just do it differently now. We talk on the phone and they tell me all about their day when they get home".

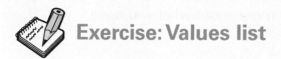

Exercise: Values list

It can be hard at first to think about what you value, especially if you feel far away or disconnected from the things, people or activities that are, or used to be, important to you. Having an idea of the things you value now can help you to regain a sense of 'you'.

There is a list of some values at the back of this book.

● Read the list and ask yourself

    ○ Which values are very important to me and my life?

    ○ Which are important to me?

    ○ Which are not so important to me?

● You may find it helpful to note down which values fall into which of the above categories.

● Remember to notice when your mind tells you where you 'should' or 'shouldn't' put a value. What does your gut feeling tell you? It can be helpful to go with your gut for this exercise. If you notice a value that used to be important to you, but you now feel disconnected from it, ask yourself

    ○ Is this value still important to me, even though it is painful to think about it? What difference would it make to me to reconnect to this? Can I work toward it?

    ○ Is this value no longer important to me? Can I let it go? What difference would that make to me and my life?

● Once you have created your 'Very Important', 'Important' and 'Not Important' lists, take a moment and pick your 'top 5' values for right now. Then circle the value which is the most important to you. Write them down below:

....

....

....

....

....

● It may be helpful to come back to this list from time to time, to check in and see if your values list and priorities are changing or staying the same.

As you do this exercise, you might notice that a value you used to prioritize now feels very difficult to connect to. It can be helpful to ask yourself if this is because the value is no longer important to you – perhaps your priorities have changed? Or is it because you feel like you have been pulled very far away from it, so that it now feels unreachable?

It may be helpful to consider if you can find different ways to reconnect to it, in ways that are manageable for you now. This can be particularly important to think about for times when you are not well or you are not physically able to do what you did before.

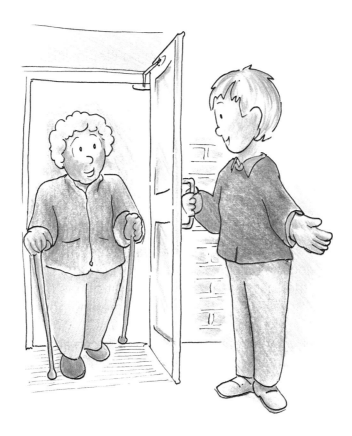

For example, if the value of 'caring' is one of your top values, you could connect to it in the following ways:

● Help out with the childcare for your grandchildren.

● Play ball and run around the garden together when they visit.

● Lie on the floor and play a quiet game together.

● Sit in the chair and read them a story.

● Speak to them on the phone or video call.

● Invite the children to sit on the bed with you and have a cuddle.

It can be painful to recognize that you cannot do things as you did before. However, finding other ways to connect to a value can still be very meaningful.

> "I used to value 'adventure'. I've been traveling and lived all over the world. I can't do this anymore and at first, I thought that meant that it's no longer important. But underneath it felt like a huge loss. Now I've realized I still do really value it; I just have to find different ways to act on it. So I helped my nephew to climb a tree for the first time … . It's not the same but I can have small moments of adventure. I can share this value with him".

Finding purpose and meaning in the face of pain

At times of pain, it is easy to feel like giving up on life, losing hope or putting your life on hold. When facing cancer, connecting to our values can remind us of the pain we are facing.

> "My cancer has come back, I'm living my worst nightmare! But I can still be me and look after myself by living the life I want to live even through treatment, with the physical challenges I face and in the limited time that I may have, no one can take that control away".

It is very difficult to get rid of this pain, but people understandably try hard to do so. For example, some people find themselves becoming more distant from the people they care about most. Acting in this way makes sense when you consider it is often the person's way of trying to avoid hurting their loved ones or the huge sense of loss about not being here in the future. However, the cost of this means missing out on the relationships that matter the most to them in the here and now.

Continuing to act on your values in the face of the pain can allow you to notice the small treasures around you that are all too easy to miss. Like small moments of joy or a sense of closeness to loved ones.

> "I don't want to think about the end of my life, but planning my funeral feels really important. I want to include songs that are meaningful for the people I love the most. It's to make sure they know how much I care about them even though I can't be there anymore".

It is easy to get caught up in thoughts that tell us it must be either the pain or purpose. Stories that tell us that we have to get rid of the pain before we can do what matters. Instead, you can show yourself kindness during the pain and have a sense of purpose, connecting to your values and finding fulfillment … if it works for you. It is never too late to make a change.

Cancer can sometimes feel like a huge wakeup call that leads you to notice that things were not working for you before the diagnosis. Or that some things no longer seem as important to you as they did before. It can lead you to find new meaning and completely change the direction of your life: you may change your job or pattern of work, develop new interests and hobbies or make changes to your relationships and friendships.

Or the changes may be much smaller but equally as meaningful, such as making friends with someone new, spending more time with your family or doing a little more of the things that you enjoy. Your values will help guide you to build a more meaningful life that works for you.

> "I'm not sure how long it took me to get back to full health, probably about three years … I don't know if I'm still the woman I was, but I do know that I'm very content with the woman I am today".

> "In a strange way I feel liberated from the things that once seemed so important".

> "Work was never really the same after this period of time off, while I owe my employers for allowing me time off, I wasn't the same person in work, it no longer was the sole purpose to my life. I'd reconnected with my wife, the kids, my wider family and friends, it was important to balance my life and my priorities".

When you can give yourself some space from the difficult thoughts and feelings and you become familiar with your most important values, then you can choose what action to take. You can choose to do something that matters and makes a difference to you.

Committed action – making life meaningful

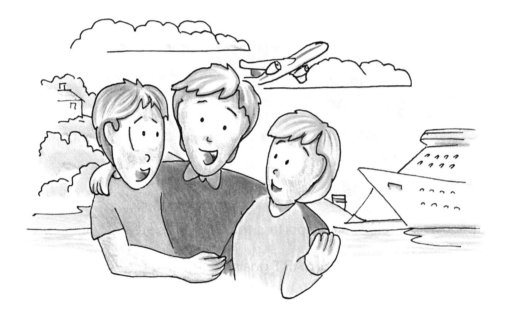

Committed action means taking action, guided by your values, even if it feels difficult or uncomfortable. It involves making a commitment to do what matters – choosing to do something which is meaningful to you. It also means standing for the things you love and value, even in the face of pain, when it gives life meaning. This can be the toughest part of living a life that matters. Committed actions are by definition toward moves.

Committed action involves:

- Making a commitment to act on a value or in a meaningful direction.

- Accepting that sometimes you may go 'off-course' (you may do this again and again and again …) and committing to getting back on track as soon as you realize you have been pulled away.

Acting on what is important to you can make it easier to realize the value of being mindful and opening up to thoughts and feelings. It can give you another focus alongside the impact of the cancer or uncertainty.

It can be useful to consider that it often is not enough just to think about doing something meaningful. It is when we take action in the service of the values that matter most to us that makes the biggest difference.

So how can we take action?

Values-based goal setting

We all set ourselves goals at times. Sometimes we are very motivated to achieve these goals. Sometimes we set goals for ourselves that we know we will never really do.

Setting yourself goals based on your values (rather than the things your mind tells you that you 'should' do) can help to motivate you. It can help you to commit to taking actions that give you a sense of meaning, purpose and fulfillment.

> "I hate radiotherapy but I can keep doing it because I want to do everything that I can to be there for my daughter's wedding".

There are six steps that can help to guide your committed action and setting yourself 'workable' goals based on your values:

1. Choose an area of your life you want to work on.

2. Think about which values are important for you in this area of your life.

3. Set yourself a **SMART** goal. **SMART** goals are

    i. **Specific:** clear and concise.

    ii. **Meaningful:** connects you to your values and sense of purpose.

iii. **Adaptive:** improves your life in some way.

iv. **Realistic:** something that is achievable.

v. **Time-framed:** you could complete this goal by a given time point.

4. Break this goal down into smaller manageable and achievable steps.

5. Ask yourself "If no one was watching or would notice, would I still do this?"

6. Identify the benefits and hurdles – what difference will this action make to you and your life? What are the barriers to this action – in the world around you as well as thoughts and feelings that you may become caught up in?

7. Make a commitment to act – write it down, tell someone else, take action.

Remember, thinking about doing something that matters often does not make much difference. It is the action of doing something that makes a difference.

It may not make a difference to anyone else if you set yourself a goal and act on it or not but it could make a big difference to you!

Often it can be helpful to ask yourself:

"What is the smallest possible, easiest step I can take toward this value in the next 24 hours?"

It can be really helpful to make sure to notice when you take a meaningful action (however small your mind tells you it is) and congratulate yourself for it. This can help you to take a moment to appreciate the difference it made to you and to help you to notice the progress you make over time. You can also check in with yourself after a week or two, notice where you started from and where you are now.

> "I've learned to appreciate doing the small things, I weed my garden and grow lovely sweet peas. My wife and I, we love beach walks and drawing in the sand".

Here are some exercises to help you to take small steps toward living the life you want to live and steering your actions according to your values. Try to remember the tips above when you complete them.

Exercise: My values-based goals

	In the next 48 hours	In the next days–weeks	In the next weeks–months	In the next months–years
Specific A clear, concrete description of what you're going to *do*				
Meaningful What value is it connecting you to?				
Adaptive What difference will it make to you and your life?				
Realistic How will you know when you've achieved it?				
Time-framed Exactly when are you going to do this?				

Barriers to action

To help you to take committed action, consider the following barriers to action and how you can overcome these:

- **Unclear or poorly set goals:** If a goal is not SMART, it can be much harder to commit to and harder to recognize when you've achieved your goal.

- **Emotional goals:** Setting yourself a goal to 'feel' a certain way is likely to keep you stuck as it is not something you can control. Focus your goal instead on acting in a certain way.

- **"I'll try, but …":** This often shows that the goal you have set is too big a step or you've set it because your mind is telling you that you 'should' do it. Is this goal connected to an important value? What difference it would make to you if you acted on it? Can you break it down into even smaller steps?

- **"But it makes me feel bad …":** Setting yourself a values-based goal may bring up pain in the short term. Would acting on this value add fulfillment, meaning or purpose to your life? If yes, are you willing to experience the difficult feelings to move closer to your chosen value?

- **"I don't know how …":** Allow yourself time to imagine what it would be like if you were living by your chosen value. What would a camera or a fly on the wall see you doing? Set yourself a small goal that takes you closer to this. You can build on this goal one step at a time.

- **"I want to stop …":** A goal that is about not doing something or doing less of something is hard to do. Instead, change it to a goal about doing something. Ask yourself, "if I was no longer doing X, Y, Z, what would I be doing with my time instead?". Make that your goal.

> "Since the cancer diagnosis, I've been eating more and more junk food. When I try to cut it out, I just crave it more. Now I've set myself the goal to eat one more portion of fruit or vegetables a day instead. I can still have chocolate as a treat and I'm valuing my health more".

Summary

Within Part 2 of this book, we have explored an ACT approach to help you to think about when you can choose to take steps toward a life that is meaningful and fulfilling, even when it feels like the cancer is pulling you away from the things that matter to you.

We have explored different techniques, including dropping anchor, mindfulness, Defusion, Expansion, Urge Surfing, self-compassion and values-based committed action.

These ideas and techniques allow you to face serious difficulties and to experience difficult thoughts and feelings without letting go of what matters most to you.

Opening up and allowing yourself to experience difficult thoughts and feelings can help you to turn toward the things you value in your life and to be the person you want to be. You can use your time, effort and energy to prioritize what is meaningful and important to you and to live a more fulfilling life despite all the hurdles that cancer throws your way.

Putting all these things together – opening up and being present, choosing a valued direction and taking action – helps you to have more tools in your toolkit to respond when life feels tough. It helps you to find more flexible ways of coping and connecting, no matter what you are facing. In other words, a helpful way to remember this is

Be present, open up, and do what matters to you.

The greater your ability to do this, the more you can choose to do the things that give you a better quality of life as well as a sense of vitality, well-being and fulfillment.

References

Ciarrochi, J., Bailey, A., & Harris, R. (2014). *The weight escape: How to stop dieting and start living*. Boston: Shambhala Publications.

Harris, R. (2017). Choice Point 2.0: A brief overview. wwww.actmindully.com.au.

Harris, R. (2018). *ACT Questions and answers*. Oakland, CA: New Harbinger Press.

Harris, R. (2019). *ACT Made Simple: An Easy-To-Read Primer on Acceptance and Commitment Therapy* (Second Edition). New Harbinger Publications.

Harris, R. (2021). The Reality Slap 2nd Edition: How to survive and thrive when life hits hard. Little, Brown Book Group.

3 Looking after yourself

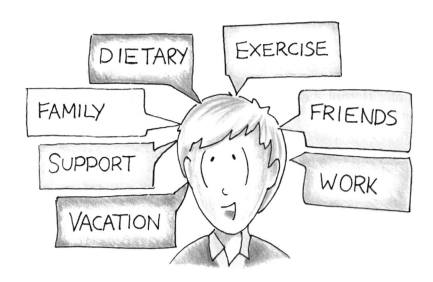

Self-care

When you are able to drop anchor and become aware of what is showing up for you in your mind and body, you have a choice about what you do in response. You can choose to do what takes you toward the things that matter to you. It may be how you want to behave toward yourself (self-care), or toward other people or what you want to do in the world according to your values.

If you have strong values about caring, your first actions may be to look after other people who are important to you. You may have forgotten how important it is to look after yourself. Perhaps you have never prioritized yourself. You might have always put the people you care about first to try to make the situation better for them and to make sure that they are OK. You may notice stories coming up, such as "that is selfish" or "I shouldn't spend time on myself" or "I am not worth it". If this is the case, you may have forgotten, or never learned, that unless you care for yourself as well you will most likely end up being too exhausted and unable to do anything for anyone or to do things that matter.

It may be helpful to think about the 'teapot analogy'. You are the teapot. Other people and activities you want to spend time doing are the cups. The tea is care. When your teapot is full, you can pour some into the cups. You can keep pouring cups of tea until your pot is empty. If you do not take the time to refill your tea pot, you will not be able to continue to pour tea. Keeping your teapot regularly topped up means you never run out of tea.

Similarly, when you are on an airplane, the safety briefing asks you to put your own oxygen mask on before you help others. This is to make sure you are safe and cared for first. Once you are safe and have the oxygen supply you need, then you are much more able to give other people the help they need.

Self-care does not have to take a long time or involve big changes. Often a few small self-care actions during a day can make a big difference to your overall sense of well-being. It is about making sure that you have the basics right first (such as routine, exercise/activity, sleep and being kinder to yourself) to help you feel more able to deal with the 'bigger' stuff you are facing.

This section talks through some important self-care ideas that you may find useful. They will hopefully help you to top up your teapot and use your tea wisely.

Helpful self-care strategies

There are a lot of different ideas within this section, which cover some of the most common difficulties that are associated with cancer and go on to provide coping strategies that may be useful. The most important thing is to try the strategies in this section that you think could be most helpful to you. You may not find them easy to use at first, so it can be helpful to pick one or two strategies and to practice them. Once you feel more confident using these, you can add in other ones if you wish.

Daily routine and activities

Routine

When you have cancer, it can feel like your life has been turned upside down. You may have many hospital appointments for treatment, tests and results. You may not be working anymore or feel unable to do your usual hobbies, activities or things for your friends and family. It may feel like everything has changed. People often do not realize how important their daily routine is in helping them feel like themselves. It can take time to adjust to the short- and long-term side effects of treatment. To balance this out, try to stick to your usual routines where possible during treatment and keep doing things you enjoy.

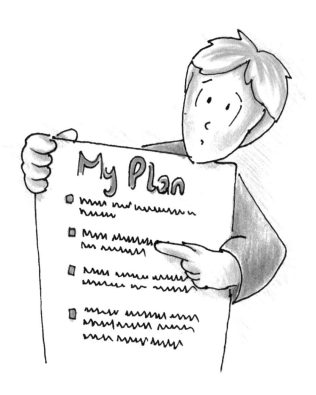

- **Make a daily plan:** When you are struggling or feeling down, you may not feel like doing anything; you have gone into 'Freeze'. You may find it hard to decide what to do each day and can end up doing very little. A good way to keep active is to make a daily plan at the start of each day or week. Here are some tips that will help this to work:

  - Begin by making a list of things you want to do (include things you enjoy doing, not just the things you feel you 'need' to do or 'should' do).

  - Try to include some physical activities since these can help to lift mood and improve sleep.

  - Mixing with friends, family and neighbors can be helpful.

  - Plan a daily action list with the easiest task first.

  - Do not aim too high, be kind to yourself, do things in small, manageable steps.

  - Work through the action list and tick off what you have done – at the end of the day you will be able to look back and recognize that you are doing things that matter.

  - If there are things you could not do, ask yourself what would make them easier? Are they really important? And if they are, what got in the way? Is there anyone you can ask to help you?

- **Do something nice:** When things are hard, you may forget the importance of doing something nice for yourself. You may also not realize the ways in which the things you have done are connected to your values and can give you a sense of well-being. The following steps can help with this:

  - On your daily action plan write down all events of the day.

  - Put a 'W' next to those which have given you a sense of well-being.

  - Put a 'V' next to those activities where you did something that was connected to your values.

  - Notice if it makes a difference to you when you have allowed yourself time for self-care activities or treated yourself to something nice.

  - Allow yourself to recognize times that you have been able to do something that matters, even if it seems small, and give yourself credit for them.

  > "I hadn't realized that I was only going to appointments then trying my hardest to do the chores and get the dinner cooked. My battery was always empty and I had no 'me' time at all. It made it so much easier to get up in the morning when I planned some time to sit in the garden and just watch the birds or to go for a drive to the beach to watch the sea".

● **Take a break:** It is normal to feel more tired than usual when going through treatment and when living with the impact of cancer. If you are finding a particular situation or task tough, drop anchor and try giving yourself some space to think about the most helpful thing you could do at that moment. You can then return to the situation and keep going if you want to do so. If you cannot move away, you can try focusing on your breathing, picturing yourself somewhere else or just have a quiet moment to yourself.

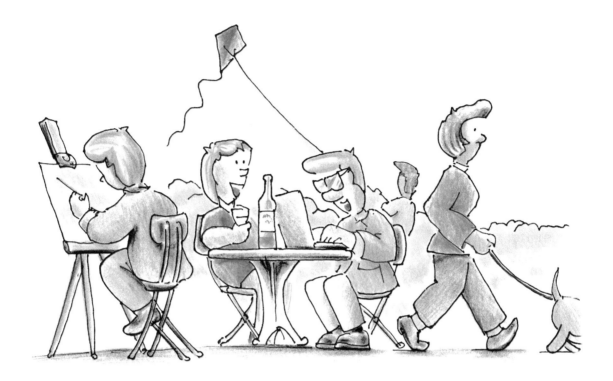

● **Reward yourself:** It is important to be kind to yourself and reward yourself for your successes – however small they seem to you. For example, getting dressed in the morning is sometimes an achievement after treatment. Recognizing this will help to build your confidence. Remember to ask for support if you need it and do things you enjoy as well.

● **It is OK to opt out:** It can be tempting to do more than you are physically able to do, just to feel like 'you' again. For example, often people feel that they must answer the phone because someone has been kind enough to call but end up feeling wiped out afterward. Only you know how you are feeling each day and whether you feel up to doing something. It is OK to say no to some things to help you to prioritize your time and energy for the things that matter most to you. You can always call the person back when you are feeling a little better.

"I just wanted to get back to normal so much. I kept pushing myself to do the shopping. My partner had been doing so much for me I just wanted to give her a break … but I ended up exhausted and all I could do was sleep afterward. She told me she was happy to do it but I felt guilty. The day I let myself stay home, we had more time to talk and laugh together".

Physical activity

In the past, people who had been diagnosed with cancer were often told to rest during treatment. However, we now know that being active can help you manage some of the side effects of cancer and/or its treatments.

There are lots of benefits to keeping active during and after cancer treatment, both for your body and your mind.

Activity can help reduce fatigue, increase your appetite, build muscle and bone strength, help your heart, keep you fit and help you maintain a healthy weight.

Activity can also help you manage stress, anxiety and low mood. There is evidence that for some people being active can reduce the risk of cancer coming back in the future.

However, the thought of becoming active can be overwhelming, particularly if you have not been active before or for some time. It may have been that this was something that was very important to you, but you feel far away from where you were before. It can be difficult to know where to start or you may worry about whether you will be able to get back to your previous activity levels.

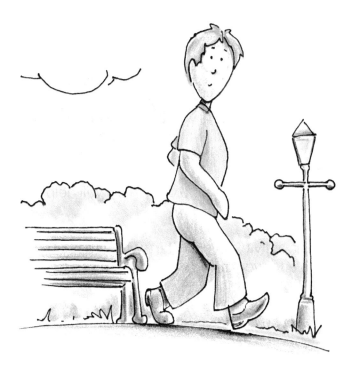

It is suggested that all adults should try and do 150 minutes (2 hours 30 minutes) of moderate-intensity activity every week. This may sound like a lot but the activity does not have to be done all at the same time.

For example, you could try 30 minutes of activity five times per week. If you are just starting to increase your activity levels or are having treatment, you may want to split this into shorter times and spread them out over the day. For example, three 10-minute sessions in one day.

It can also be hard to know how intense your activity levels need to be. As a rule, moderate-intensity activity should make you feel a little warmer, make your heart beat a little quicker and your breathing a little faster, but you can still hold a conversation while you do it.

Tips for getting active and staying active

There are many ways that you can become more active. Here are some ideas:

- Try not to sit and lie down for a long time in the day – do small amounts of activity throughout the day.

- Build activity into things you do every day. These things count toward your daily amount of activity. They can help your health in the same way as swimming, running and cycling. You can build small moments of activity into your daily routine. For example:

    o Doing some housework.

    o Take the stairs rather than the lift.

    o Get off the bus a stop early and walk the rest of the journey home.

    o Do some gardening.

    o Walk or cycle to places instead of driving when possible.

- Make goals that you can achieve. If you have never run before or for a long time, start by building up to running for five minutes. As the activity gets easier, set a new goal.

- Write down when you do an activity in a diary. This will help you to remain motivated and to see what you have achieved.

- Gradually build up your activity levels. Start with small amounts of activity, slowly increasing it over days and weeks.

- Do something that you enjoy. You are more likely to stick to your activity plan and achieve your goals if you do an activity that you find fun.

- Trying a new activity or changing your activities will help to keep your interest and enjoyment.

- Set yourself a series of small achievable steps. Remind yourself that even trying to do some activity is a toward move. Reward yourself when you achieve each step.

    o For example, if you want to start walking and haven't left the house for a while, start by walking to the front door. Then to the end of the garden path. Build up slowly each day until you can walk to the end of the road. Allow yourself to take rests along the way. You can keep adding a little bit extra in as you feel able to.

● Try to be kind to yourself if you are having a bad day, or if you are not going as quickly as you would like. You can get back on track when you are having a better day.

● You do not have to do it alone – asking family or friends to do some activities with you can help to keep you motivated. You may also want to think about joining a sports club or group.

● Remember that you can ask for advice from your medical team.

"I used to love mountain biking and I miss it so much. I can't wait to get back on my bike. I also don't know if I'll be able to again. Having help from the physio has helped me to get up and about again. It is a long road but I'm a step closer".

"My recovery from surgery is taking much longer than I had hoped for but building up my activity made me feel like I was getting somewhere. I felt a bit more like me again".

Relaxation

Just as important as increasing our activity levels is making sure we have time when we can relax.

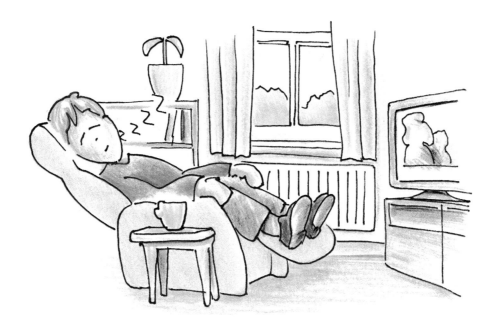

Relaxation can help us to:

● Self-care

● Reduce aches and pains

- Lower blood pressure

- Increase energy levels

- Improve sleep

- Improve our sense of well-being

How can I learn to relax?

The ability to relax is not always something which comes naturally – it is a skill which must be practiced. You will likely have experienced feelings of relaxation in the past. For example, when sitting in the garden, listening to music or walking along a beach. You can learn to recall these feelings and to relax more deeply by practicing relaxation techniques.

There are various types of relaxation including:

- **Breathing exercises:** slowing your breathing rate to a comfortable, calming or soothing pace. It can help to count your breath in and out, taking a pause after each in and out breath.

- **Muscle relaxation:** focusing on and relaxing the muscles within different areas of your body in turn.

- **Guided imagery:** involves the creation of a relaxing image, e.g. a beach, waterfall or safe place in your mind and using the five senses to help you to build a sense of relaxation.

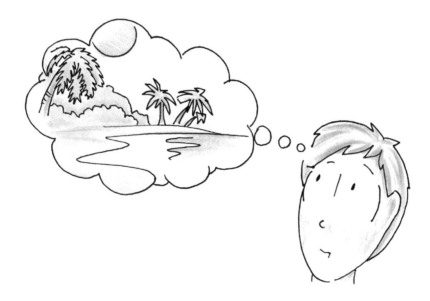

Different methods suit different people. The important thing is to find out which ones help you.

Relaxation can be done alone or in a group. Like any new skill, learning to relax deeply takes time and practice. Some days you will find it easier to relax than others.

Tips for relaxation:

- Plan your relaxation.

- Find a quiet place where you will not be disturbed.

- Make sure you are comfortable on a supportive chair or bed or lying on the floor – your whole body from your head to your feet needs to be supported.

- Make sure you are warm enough and not in a draft. You may find having a blanket is helpful.

- Just notice how your body is feeling.

- You may experience sensations of floating, heaviness, warmth or tingling. This is quite normal.

- Following relaxation, give yourself time to become alert, stretch and get up slowly before resuming your daily activities.

> "Just sitting for five minutes a day and focusing on my breathing made such a difference".

> "When things were tough I would take myself to my favorite place ... the beach ... hearing the waves and feeling the sun ... even when I just imagined myself there it was strangely calming ... the only downside was I was always left wanting an ice cream!"

Within the Resources section at the back of this book, we have included websites and apps that have examples of different relaxation methods. There are also relaxation exercises on the website link given in Part 4 of this book.

 ## KEY MESSAGES

- Create new routines in your life and make daily plans. Make sure that you plan to do something nice for yourself every day.

- Recognize and reward yourself for your achievements as small as they might feel.

- Give yourself permission to say no to yourself and other people.

- Increasing activity levels slowly can help with physical and psychological well-being. Reward yourself when you have met your goals.

- Relaxation can increase our sense of well-being. It is just as important as activity.

Stay connected

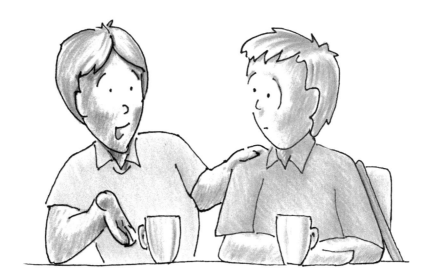

Living with cancer can sometimes make you feel very alone, as if no one truly understands what you are going through. One of the reasons that this book includes the words of people affected by cancer and their family or friends is to help you feel connected to others – to help you notice you are not so isolated or on your own.

Remember that we are all struggling with similar thoughts and feelings. Just hearing that other people have the same concerns and worries can be very helpful in dropping the struggle and giving yourself permission to be 'kind to yourself'.

Having a support network that you trust can be an important part of self-care too. It gives you someone to turn to for help or comfort. If you can, try to stay connected with groups you already belong to, including your friends and family.

This may be difficult at times due to the stories that come up, such as "I am no fun" or "I don't have the energy to talk" or "I don't want them to ask me questions". Sometimes talking to friends or family can feel hard, as you may be worried about upsetting them.

"I can't let my family know that I am not coping … I am meant to be the strong one … everyone comes to me! How can I be the one to cause them worry by telling them I'm frightened".

"Everyone told me not to tell my mum as she was too frail … I listened for a while but felt that I was keeping a secret … and I missed my mum looking out for me … she was upset when I told her of course but she told me that it would have hurt her more if I had kept it from her … she said that she knew something was wrong".

"It was really important for me to have control over who knew at work; it is my business and I need it to stay that way".

We hope that the skills you have learned in Part 2, such as how to defuse, expand and then to do something that matters, will help you to be with the people that you love and who love you.

You may have also noticed that your relationship has changed with some friends and members of your family. You may be closer to some people but feel more distant from others.

"My closest friend broke my heart, she just stopped calling, stopped asking me out with the group".

"I never thought my neighbor Sam would be the rock that they have been; we went from friendly acquaintances to friends for life".

Remember, that friends and family who are not familiar with the ideas and skills in this book may be hooked into trying to avoid painful thoughts and feelings about what has happened to you and how it is affecting them. They may not know what they can do to help. As a result, they may not return your calls, be too busy to meet up or not feel able to talk about what you are going through. Your overly helpful mind may be shouting very loudly that "they don't care about you", leaving you feeling sad and maybe angry. When these thoughts and feelings show up, drop anchor, make space and then do something that takes you toward the relationship that you would like with them.

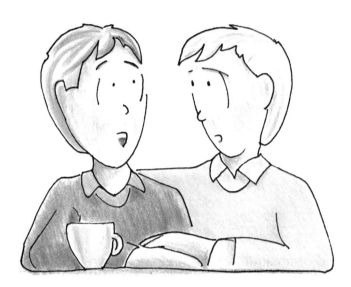

For example, you could let them know that they don't have to try to make it better for you, just spending time together is important. It can help to tell them that some days you might want to talk about the cancer and on other days you don't. Or perhaps you could just let them know you are missing them.

You may also make new friends through treatment or from new activities that you try. It can be hard to try new things at first; you may not know what to expect or you may feel very worried about getting upset or embarrassed. Hopefully, using some of your new skills will help you to unhook, take that step and go to a group or class. Try to notice who looks and sounds friendly and take steps toward connecting with them.

There may be support groups available where you can talk to people who have had similar experiences and concerns. There are also now more and more internet-based groups. There are also lots of websites and helplines you can access for more support and information. You can ask your healthcare team about how to find groups for your age, gender or cancer type. Many groups are organized locally, so we have included some useful places for you to start to find one that interests you in the Resources section.

"By far the greatest benefit for me [of cancer] has been the friends I've made along the way. People from all walks of life providing a strong network of friendship and support, most definitely the best medicine there is!"

 ## KEY MESSAGES

- At times of difficulty, it is important to have a social network around you.

- This can help you to share your concerns and to seek help and comfort from people you trust.

- It can be hard talking about what you're going through but this can also help you to feel closer.

- You may find that your relationships change, and this can be painful, it is important to look after yourself if this happens.

- It can be helpful to connect to new people who understand what it is like to be affected by cancer.

Thinking strategies

Self-talk

When we are worried or anxious, we often believe we cannot cope. Our minds often come up with critical stories. Remind yourself to drop anchor and acknowledge what has shown up. You may have thoughts like "I can't do this" or "things always go wrong". When you become aware of what these thoughts are telling you, you can thank your mind for trying to help and then use coping statements such as:

- "That's the 'I can't do it' story".

- "There is anxiety".

- "I have got through it before".

- "This will pass".

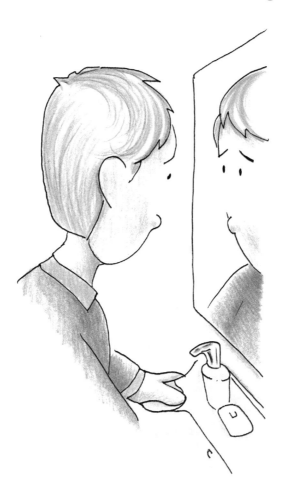

Self-talk with a kind voice. You could try a simple Defusion strategy. Remind yourself that you can unhook from the stream of thoughts, feelings and sensations that come up.

This can help to boost your confidence and help you feel able to acknowledge difficult thoughts or feelings and focus on doing what is important to you.

If you continue to struggle, use the other Defusion or Expansion skills and notice what your thoughts and feelings are trying to tell you. You can choose whether you want to be kind to yourself and use self-care or do a different 'toward move' based on your values that are coming up. Talk kindly to yourself as you do so.

Balanced thinking

When your mind is telling you stories or trying to solve problems, it often forgets to use all the information that is available. It hooks you into the scariest information and trying to find a potential situation to the threat. It is trying to be helpful and keep you safe. When this happens, sometimes a useful technique to try is called 'balancing'. When you have an unbalanced thought, you can try to balance it out by saying a more accurate and helpful statement to yourself.

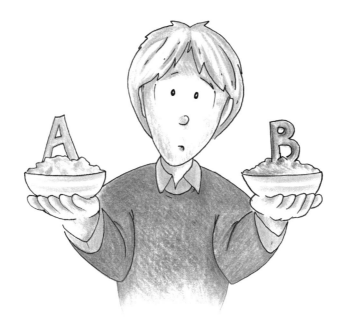

For example, the thought "My results will be bad" could be balanced with "If the cancer has come back, my doctor said they would have another treatment plan to sort it".

Note: This technique does not aim to get rid of the unhelpful thought, it just helps you to consider another perspective too.

 ### Exercise: The double column technique

Another thing you could do is write down your thought in one column and in an opposite column, write down a more balanced thought for each one.

Like this:

John has not called; he does not want to talk to me anymore because he is bored by 'cancer'.	He is very busy and thinks I am doing better than I was last week. So, he thinks he doesn't need to worry about me.

You can try this for yourself in the space below:

It is important to remember that our mind is trying to be helpful. We are not trying to persuade it to say something positive or argue against it or silence it. We are just trying to be more aware of the 'bigger picture' and do something that takes us toward our values.

KEY MESSAGES

- Talking to yourself kindly is an important part of self-care.

- When you notice your thoughts are unbalanced, it can be helpful to step back and take a wider perspective.

- Writing down balanced, alternative thoughts can help you with this.

Taking control (when it is workable)

Distraction

Just as the name suggests, distraction is anything you do to temporarily take your attention off a painful thought and feeling. You may have used it a lot when painful thoughts and feelings have shown up or when you have been acting in autopilot mode. A key part of the above explanation of distraction is the word "temporarily". Has distraction worked for you in the long term? Most people notice that distraction only tends to work for a short while, eventually the thoughts or feelings come back.

If you are using distraction all the time to try and get rid of thoughts and feelings, then it is most likely to be an 'away move'. However, there are times when distraction can be a toward move. When going through treatment such as radiotherapy or chemotherapy, it can be particularly hard to just get through each treatment or test. Each appointment is a 'short-term' event. Each short-term appointment takes you closer to your longer-term goal of completing the course of treatment (if you choose this is the best course of action for you).

In this situation, distraction can be described as a 'toward move'; i.e. distraction is helping you to get through each treatment, giving the strong thoughts and feelings time to settle down and helping you to stay in the situation.

> "If I talk to myself during my scan by counting down from 300, I can get through it".

How to distract yourself

The most helpful distractions are often connected to doing things that matter to you as they grab your attention; there are several things you can try to distract yourself. Listed below are some examples:

- Count backward from a large number by sevens or some other number (for example, 856, 849, 842, 835, etc.).

- Take part in a fun and challenging game that requires some level of attention, such as a crossword puzzle or sudoku.

- Focus your attention on your environment – name all the colors in the room or try to memorize and recall all the objects that you see around you.

- Do something creative, like drawing a picture or building a model.

- Read a good book or watch a funny film.

- Call or write a letter to someone you care about.

- Do some 'window-shopping' online.

- Take part in a self-soothing strategy, such as deep breathing, listening to music or a podcast.

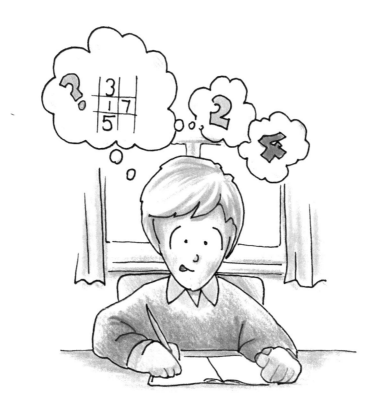

 ### Exercise: Finding your own distractions

Try to come up with your own list of distraction activities that you can use when you experience a strong feeling or thought that is hard to cope with in the moment. The more you can come up with, the more flexible you can be in deciding which is the best activity for the situation you are in. Over time, when you strengthen your skills in 'Urge Surfing', you may choose to use that skill instead of distraction.

You can write down some of your ideas here:

....

....

....

....

....

Problem solving

Just like distraction, problem solving can be both a toward and away move. It can help you work out what you need to do to take you toward the life that you would like to live. On the other hand, your overly helpful mind can keep telling you to use problem solving to find a solution without realizing that the problem is unsolvable (an away move). The trick is to choose to use problem solving when it is helpful and notice when you are stuck or going round in circles.

It is important to note that the impact of cancer can have a significant effect on your ability to solve problems. It can feel harder to do if you now have difficulties with concentration and memory.

You also may not have as many practical resources or as much physical strength, which can limit the number of possible solutions. You also may be faced with problems that you have never had to work through before because of coping with the impact of cancer.

"When I heard about six weeks of radiotherapy, I panicked about how I was going to get there every day and get back in time to pick up the children from school".

"I can't get in and out of the bath at the moment, I am so exhausted and in discomfort all the time".

You may find it helpful to remind yourself of the key steps in problem solving to help you manage some of these additional challenges:

Solving difficult problems

Step 1: I think I have a problem

- Pay attention to your feelings: as you now know difficult feelings are often trying to tell you something that matters to you is threatened (e.g. your ability to care for a loved one, your physical well-being). Paying attention to these feelings, instead of ignoring them, can help you to think about the problem that you are facing. You can then give yourself space to think about any things you can do to help to solve the problem.

  - For example, if you are worried about having too many side effects of treatment, it can be helpful to talk to your medical team about this. They can tell you whether they can change your treatment plan to ease the side effects, rather than just 'putting up with them'.

- Make a list: Write out a list of the problems you need to think through before they turn into bigger problems. Some problems seem to stick around. Others seem to go away, but they may pop up again later.

Step 2: What is the problem?

- You cannot solve a problem until you know what the problem is. To do that, ask yourself these questions:

    ○ What is the situation right now? What is making me feel upset?

    ○ What would I like the situation to be? How would things be if I were not upset?

    ○ What are the obstacles? What is standing between me and my ideal situation?

- Be as specific as possible: if your definition of the problem is vague, it is hard to know where your solution should start. For example, it would be hard to solve a money problem if you say, "I have money problems". A more precise definition might be, "I don't have enough money to pay the minimum mortgage payment".

- Stick to the facts: try not to put opinions in your definition, only facts.

- Don't be too narrow: when you define the problem too narrowly, it's harder to come up with solutions.

    ○ For example, you would like to travel this summer, but it is hard to get reasonably priced insurance after a cancer diagnosis. A narrow definition might be, "How can I get enough money to pay for insurance?". A better definition might be, "How can I travel this summer within my budget?". When you define your problem like this, buying insurance is only one of many solutions. Your solutions could also include getting a deal on a local holiday, taking a coach rather than a plane or going to see friends.

Step 3: How will I know when I get there?

- Choose a goal for your problem. The SMART principle may help you set goals. (Notice that SMART for problem solving is different to SMART for committed action):

    ○ Goals should be:

        • Specific

        • Measurable

        • Attainable

        • Realistic and

        • Time-limited

- For example, "not having money problems" is not a good goal statement because it doesn't tell you what to do and when to do it. A helpful goal statement may be "I am going to apply for the benefits I am entitled to".

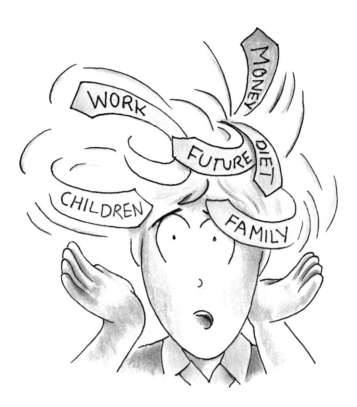

Step 4: What are some possible solutions?

● When faced with a problem, you have learned that the first solutions that automatically appear in your mind are not always the best. They are often just trying to get rid of the threat in the here and now and not thinking about whether it would be a helpful thing to do in the long term.

● It's easier to find a good solution that takes you toward the life you would like when you have a lot of solutions to choose from.

   ○ Write out at least three or four solutions – the more the better.

   ○ Notice when your mind is telling you judgment stories and you get hooked into the thoughts and feelings. This is not the time to decide whether your solutions are good or not.

   ○ Variety: Come up with lots of different kinds of solutions.

      ● For example, if your solutions to money problems include borrowing from your friends, your parents or your sibling, you have come up with three solutions that all involve the same idea: borrowing money. Instead, it can help you to have many different types of solutions, such as selling some of your unwanted possessions or applying for a grant.

   ○ You are more likely to think of new solutions if you also include some wild and creative ones.

- Ask others for help.

- Get new ideas from friends, family or professionals.

Step 5: What is the best solution?

- Always pick the best solution for you – the perfect solution rarely exists. The key is to pick the solution that has the most benefits and takes you toward a valued life. There will probably be some negatives or consequences to any solution. Use the following questions as a guide to pick the best solution.

- Will this solution help me reach my goals and solve my problem? If a solution does not solve the problem, it is probably not the best choice.

- How much time and effort does this solution involve? Solutions that take up too much time and energy may not be the best choice, especially if you cannot realistically carry them out.

- Does this solution have more benefits than costs? When you look at costs and benefits, it is a good idea to think about how a solution will affect you and others – both now and in the future.

- How will I feel if I choose this solution? You may come up with solutions that could solve the problem very well. If you think that the solution will make you feel terrible, it may not be the best choice at this time. However, if something is painful in the short term but helpful in the long term, it could be worth considering if it takes you toward what matters to you in life.

- Most importantly, ask yourself if I 'solve' this problem, will it take me closer to the life that I would like to live based on my values?

Step 6: Put your solution into action

- After you have picked a solution, you need to make a plan of action. Write down the steps it will take to carry out your solution. You are more likely to act if you know exactly what you need to do.

  "I was panicking that I would never be able to pay all my bills and just buried my head in the sand … I sat down with an advisor and we worked it through in steps … it still wasn't easy … but my head was back above water and I could focus on the important stuff … treatment".

  "My head was spinning about how to manage childcare and treatment … it wasn't until my nurse said have you tried problem-solving that I could see the wood for the trees … it's strange that when you're overwhelmed you don't think of using something that you do every day".

Step 7: Check up on your progress

- It is a good idea to track how well your solution is working. If your problem is resolving itself, be sure to reward yourself for a job well done.

- If your solution is taking you away from being you and living a meaningful life, you can check to see what might be wrong. Remember, even the best plans do not always work as expected. If your solution does not seem to be working, ask yourself the following questions:

    ○ Did I define my problem correctly?

    ○ Were my goals unrealistic?

    ○ Was there a better solution?

    ○ Did I carry out the solution properly?

- You may need to go through these steps more than once until you have a satisfactory solution. This is normal – especially for more difficult problems.

 KEY MESSAGES

- It can be helpful to distract yourself to get through a short-term, unpleasant situation, such as treatment, if this helps you to get to where you need to be in the longer term.

- Problems can impact on our well-being.

- You may not know what the problem is but know that there is something wrong.

- We automatically do what we have always done in the past to solve the problem – this may not be the most helpful solution.

- Problem solving can help find a good solution that fits with your life and gives you a sense of control.

Managing some common problems

Some problems like fatigue, pain, eating problems and sleep difficulties affect many people with cancer. Below we have provided some specific information on how to manage these issues.

Sleep

When you are having treatment for cancer, you can often find that your sleep can be affected. Sleep problems can also occur for several reasons: certain factors related to getting older, medical reasons, emotional reasons, unhelpful surroundings or disruptive sleep routines.

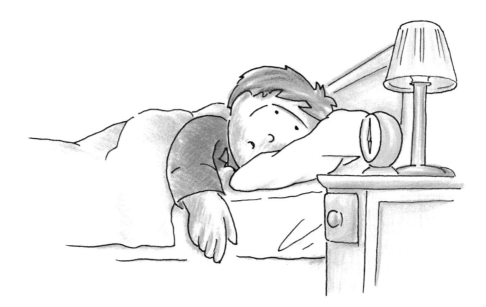

There are different sorts of sleep problems: getting to sleep, staying asleep, waking too early or poor-quality sleep. It is also possible to think that you have a sleep problem when in fact you are still getting enough sleep, but it is different from what you expect to have.

Everyone needs a different amount of sleep to experience a sense of well-being. If you are not getting enough sleep, it can affect you psychologically and emotionally. You can end up noticing feelings of anxiety, frustration and low mood with a sense of hopelessness.

"There is nothing worse than lying awake at 2am when the rest of the world is sleeping and you're trying to deal with your darkest thoughts".

"I used to dread night times; I was all alone with my thoughts with no chance to escape".

"When things got tough, I would go to bed and go to sleep, and hope things were better when I woke up; it sometimes worked but not often".

You may have noticed that bedtime and at night is the time when you are most likely to be overwhelmed by your thoughts and feelings. Your mind is using the time when things are quieter to make sure you are listening to what it is saying about the potential threats that could come up.

When you feel threatened, your body is doing its job by staying awake. Remember that your body was designed to keep you safe and go into fight, flight or freeze mode when faced with a threat. It is not a good idea to go to sleep when faced with a tiger! It becomes even trickier as the fact that you cannot get to sleep also becomes a threat. Before you know it, your mind becomes even busier and you are even more awake.

Overcoming your sleep problems

One of the first steps in overcoming sleep difficulties is finding any possible causes and trying to look for solutions.

- Is sleeping your main problem?

- Is there another problem which may be causing you to have difficulty sleeping (e.g. worry)?

- If there is another problem, is there anything you can do about the problem?

You may find that getting help in another area has a knock-on effect on your sleeping. Your sleep may well right itself if you can solve some of your other problems. However, you may have got into some 'bad' habits which are not helping you get off to sleep.

> "If I have had a bad day, I just go to bed so it is over but then I don't see the kids and feel guilty. I then sleep worse at night too".

The following simple checklist of helpful sleep habits may help.

- **Tackle the worry:** If you worry about not getting enough sleep, then this can keep you awake longer – remind yourself that you may be getting enough, but it's just less than you expect. Thank your mind for trying to be helpful. You can try Defusion or Mindfulness exercises from Part 2 to acknowledge and let go of the worries too. Some people find writing down the worries during the day can be useful.

> "I used to worry that if I didn't sleep enough, I wouldn't be able to function … I remind myself that I might not be at my best but I can still get through".

- **Avoid naps:** If possible, don't take naps during the day to catch up. This will affect your natural sleep rhythm and can add to the problem.

- **Surroundings:** Go through this basic check list and see whether there are any simple changes you can make:

  o Noise (too noisy, too quiet?)

  o Light (too light, too dark?)

  o Comfort of mattress (too hard, too soft?)

  o Temperature of room (too hot, too cold?)

  o If you have a partner, are they keeping you awake?

- **Cigarettes:** Smoking last thing at night can keep you awake as nicotine is a stimulant. If you do smoke, try to have your last cigarette at least four hours before bedtime.

- **Food and drink:** Anything that contains caffeine taken near to bedtime will reduce the quality of sleep. Examples include coffee, tea, hot chocolate, cola and chocolate. It is best not to have any of these things within four hours of bedtime.

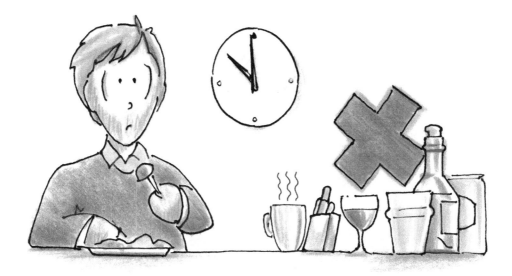

- **Medicines and other drugs:** Some drugs can affect sleep because they are stimulants. Check with your doctor if your medicines can affect sleep. While sleeping tablets can help in the short term, in the longer term they can cause sleep problems as they interfere with the quality of sleep and can alter sleep patterns. It is best to take these only for very short periods. You can discuss this with your GP.

- **Alcohol:** While people often feel sleepy after drinking a lot of alcohol, the quality of your sleep is affected. It is best to avoid drinking large amounts of alcohol close to bedtime if you are having sleep problems.

- **Consistency:** Going to bed and getting up at roughly the same time is helpful to set your natural body clock. Set an alarm if you need to.

  "I used to turn off my alarm in the middle of the night if I couldn't sleep …
  I thought a lie in would be OK … in the end I was awake all night and then
  sleeping until the afternoon … it took three weeks of using an alarm to get
  me back on track".

- **Pre-sleep routine:** Try to use the hour before going to bed to unwind and prepare for sleep (e.g. have a bath and get into pajamas or read your favorite book).

  "I was in my pajamas all day after radiotherapy for comfort … now I get
  dressed into comfy clothes in the day and change into my PJs before bed
  … it has made a huge difference to my sleep … who knew that sort of stuff
  mattered!"

- **Tiredness:** This may seem obvious but do not go to bed until you feel sleepy.

- **Activity:** Gradually increase your daytime activity and exercise, but do not exercise too near bedtime.

- **Get up:** If you have not fallen asleep within 30 minutes – get up and have a malty drink. Listen to relaxing music, read a relaxing book or watch something boring on TV until you feel sleepy.

● **Bed for sleep:** Make sure your bed is associated with sleep. For example, do not watch TV, eat and talk on the telephone in bed. The only exceptions to this are reading books and making love, which can in fact help. If your mind is hooking you into nicer stories and memories, it is OK to listen to these as they may help you to drift off.

> "My bed was a place to escape from the world … but when I couldn't sleep my bed felt like a torture device … simply moving to a comfy chair in my bedroom means I get me time. I don't have to be in bed when I don't need to sleep … and I can sleep at night".

Coping with fatigue and pain

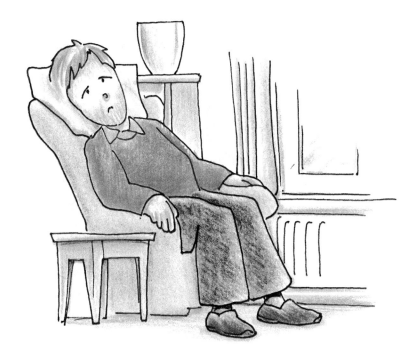

If you are feeling fatigued or in pain, it is important to let your medical team or GP know so they can support you and check if there is anything they can help you with.

> "I was spending more time in bed and journeys to and from the hospital were taking longer. It was taking longer for my wife to get me out of bed, to get me ready for the journey and then the journey itself would take longer as I constantly felt sick".

The following strategies can also help you to feel more able to do what matters when you are fatigued or in pain:

● **Exercise:** This can seem exhausting. However, small amounts of regular, gentle physical activity may help to relieve the symptoms of fatigue or pain by boosting your energy levels, mood and fitness. Examples of helpful activities include

  ○ Shopping, cooking, cleaning or gardening.

  ○ Walking, swimming, T'ai chi or yoga.

- **Diet:** Eat a well-balanced diet and drink plenty of liquids.

- **Avoid reliance on stimulants and supplements:** These include caffeine, alcohol, nicotine-based products, refined sugars and non-prescribed food supplements.

- **Prioritize:** Find a balance between what you want and need to do:

  o Does it all need to be done?

  o Does it need to be done by you?

  o Try and treat yourself to doing things you normally enjoy too.

- **Plan:** Write a list. What time of day are your energy levels highest? Keep an energy diary to assist you. Try to get a balance of activities across the day (rather than a boom-bust pattern where you do lots and then crash afterward.

- **Pace:** Be kind yourself and think about the time it takes to do tasks

  o Allow extra time to get things done.

  o Always stop before you are overtired.

  o Balance your day between activity and rest.

  o Break tasks down into smaller tasks and take regular breaks.

  "I kept trying to cook dinner all in one go because that's how I used to do it. Now I sit down to chop the vegetables in the morning. I get the rest of the ingredients and pans ready in the afternoon. Then I can just focus on cooking in the evening".

- **Give yourself permission to do things differently:** Learn to say "no" and tell others how you are feeling.

- **Position:** Make everyday tasks easier.

  o Can you sit instead of standing?

  o Reduce bending, reaching, walking or pulling by rearranging your environment.

- **Pain Medications:** Often people do not like taking too many tablets or medications. To help you cope with pain, it is important to take any medications you are prescribed as the directions tell you to do. This helps to keep your baseline level of pain as low as possible and to tackle any flare-ups that you experience.

Coping with eating difficulties

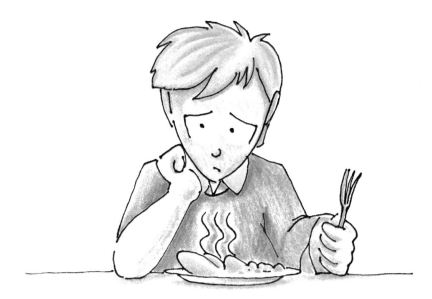

Cancer and the treatment can affect your appetite, your taste buds and can sometimes cause nausea and vomiting. This can make even the thought of eating very stressful. You may be told that it is important to keep eating during treatment, but it may feel like the last thing you want to do. It can be really helpful to speak to your dietitian or medical team for ideas and support.

"When I was diagnosed the nurse told me to eat anything and everything; healthy eating went out the window".

"I couldn't eat a thing, the thought of food made me feel sick. Nothing tasted right and my mouth hurt".

"Prior to radiotherapy starting, I was told I would lose my sense of taste – everything would taste like cardboard. Straight away after that very first session my sense of taste disappeared. I remember vividly sitting down at home tucking into a couple of fried eggs on toast and ... nothing. It looked the same as always, it smelt the same as always, but it tasted awful".

There are different types of eating difficulties that people experience following cancer. This section will give you some ideas about how to manage these things.

● **Eating when you do not feel hungry:** You may lose your appetite during your treatment due to the medicines, anxiety, worry or a combination of these.

○ Try and have three meals and two or three snacks a day. If you cannot manage three big meals, perhaps try having smaller meals more often during the day.

○ Prepare meals when you feel well enough and store them in your freezer to use when you feel ill.

○ Take a short walk before meals as exercise can stimulate your appetite.

- **Eating when your taste changes:** Your sense of taste may have changed due to the medication you are having or the treatment. This can reduce your enjoyment of eating and drinking.

  - It is very important that you keep your mouth clean. Brush your teeth before and after you eat, or at least three times a day. Brush your tongue as well if it is not sore. Use a mouthwash suggested by your nurse or radiographer. Change your toothbrush regularly (every 12 weeks).

  - If red meat tastes unpleasant, try chicken, fish, milk, cheese, beans or nuts.

  - Oranges, pineapple and lemon fruits or juices will freshen your mouth. Sip a glass before your meal and have some fruit after your meal.

  - Sugar-free chewing gum can improve the freshness of your mouth.

  - Allow your food to cool a little. Cold foods may taste better than hot.

  - Savory foods may be better than sweet foods.

  - If foods taste bland, try adding sauce to them or herbs and spices to flavor your food.

  - If you have a metal taste in your mouth while eating, try using a plastic utensil.

  - If you find any foods unpleasant, go back and retry them at a later stage as your taste may have returned.

- **Eating when you have nausea and vomiting:** You might experience nausea and vomiting due to your illness or treatment. To look after yourself through and after treatment, it can be helpful to find ways to eat something. Here are some ideas to help:

  - Eat small, frequent meals – start with small amounts and slowly increase the size of the portion.

  - If you feel sick in the morning, eat something before you get out of bed. Try plain biscuits, dry toast or crackers.

  - Keep meals dry, do not add gravy or sauces to your food and drink after your meal rather than with your food. Note: if you have had treatment for head and neck cancer, this is not a useful strategy.

  - Fizzy drinks, especially ginger ale and soda water can help nausea.

  - Posture can be important – try to remain upright while eating and after your meal.

  - Ask your doctor about medication to help with nausea and vomiting. If the nausea or vomiting lasts longer than three days, it is important to tell your doctor or nurse.

  - Bring your awareness into the room around you when you are eating, rather than on the food; watch TV, chat with friends or family, listen to your favorite music or radio show.

- **Eating to cope with difficult thoughts and feelings:** You may find yourself eating for comfort when you are not hungry, or as a distraction from difficult thoughts and feelings. This may include eating unhealthy things. It can also make you feel 'bad' after the initial distraction from distress and feeling of comfort has worn off. Difficult thoughts and feelings are a common eating trigger. It may help to track your eating habits in a journal. Note down what showed up when you reached for a snack. What thoughts, feelings and physical sensations did you notice? It may help you make a connection you had not seen before, like the fact that you eat when you are lonely or angry. Next time you notice this feeling, try to use some of the ideas in Part 2 of this book, such as Defusion, Expansion or Urge Surfing. You could also look for a different outlet, such as calling a friend when you are lonely or punching a pillow when you are angry or stressed.

- **Eating out of boredom:** For many, eating seems like a good solution when there is nothing better to do. If boredom is a trigger for your emotional eating, have a list of other things you can do to keep yourself busy and entertained when you don't have much on.

- **Eating because you are tired:** When you are feeling low in energy, it can be easy to reach for food, especially sugary treats. But that sugar rush might be followed by an even worse crash. Instead, take a walk, head outside for some fresh air and natural light or drink a glass of cold water.

- **If you eat for reasons other than being hungry:** Check in with yourself. Knowing what true hunger feels like can help you recognize when you are eating for other reasons. You can use the ideas in this book to unhook from these in the future. If you can't avoid the specific triggers that cause you to eat when you're not hungry – and there's no way to avoid them all – knowing the strategies above will help and give you a sense of control over the choices that you make with food.

 KEY MESSAGES

- The right amount of sleep for you can help you feel that you can cope physically and psychologically.

- Strategies to help you have a good sleep routine and to let go of worries can help you to improve your quality of sleep over time.

- It is important to plan, pace and prioritize the activities that matter to you when you are coping with pain and fatigue.

- Being kind to yourself can be particularly helpful when you are facing these difficulties.

- Cancer treatment can get in the way of you eating well. Recognizing why you are having difficulties with eating or how you are using eating as a coping strategy can help you find other ways that work for you.

Summary

Within this part of the book, we have explored several ways in which you can learn to deal with common difficulties that often come up alongside cancer and treatment. It may also help you to think about ways in which you can 'top up your tea pot'.

You may already be using some of these ideas. Or they may all be new to you. The key is to start with the ones that you think will be most effective at taking you toward a meaningful life, despite the cancer. It is important to consider which ideas may help you to care for your own needs – to help you to maximize the energy and time you have to do what matters most to you.

It can feel overwhelming to try too many new things at once. Be kind to yourself, start small and practice the new skills until you feel comfortable and confident using them. If you find that something you try keeps on being unhelpful, give yourself permission to let it go and try something else. You can add new techniques into your routine gradually over time.

4 Making a difference

This last part summarizes and brings together what the book has covered. It aims to helps you to think about the things you want to keep doing, things you may choose to hold onto a little less tightly and new ideas you may wish to try. This book gives you ideas you can use to help you to continue to look after yourself and live your life in a meaningful and fulfilling way, despite the cancer.

It may feel like a lot to take in, so you may choose to dip in and out or come back to sections.

Remember, there is no right or wrong way to cope or be. The Acceptance and Commitment Therapy (ACT) approach used within this book may help you to add more tools into your toolkit, to help you feel that you have more choice over what you do and to be more flexible in your approach to painful thoughts, images, feelings, sensations, memories or situations.

Below are some exercises to help you think about what could be most important or helpful for you to try, to help you remember what you have learned and to commit to doing what matters most to you.

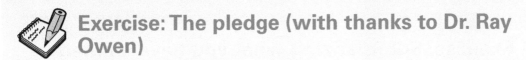 **Exercise: The pledge (with thanks to Dr. Ray Owen)**

To help you to pull together everything you have learned, it may help you to make the following pledge to yourself.

This pledge is designed to help you think about:

- What you want to do,

- Why it is important,

- What difference it makes to you and your life

- And also the painful thoughts and feelings, which may show up when you do so because you care.

Remember, sometimes the most important things we do are not always the easiest to do. We do these things because they matter. There is no guarantee that what you do will make a difference for anyone else, but it could make a difference to you. It is also important to remind yourself you matter … you deserve care and self-care too!

I will do: (what action?)

....

....

....

in the service of: (which value(s)?)

....

....

....

and am willing to experience: (which thoughts, feelings, sensations?)

....

....

....

if that's what it takes!

Exercise: Summarizing what you have learned

Thinking about your relationship to your thoughts and feelings, what have you taken away from this book at this point in time?

....

....

....

Thinking about your values and actions, what have you taken away from this book now?

....

....

....

Imagine you were to come across your future self in a couple of months or years and you wanted to remind yourself of the personally meaningful parts of this book – what would you say?

....

....

....

Moving forward

In this book, we have described what it may feel like to live with the uncertainty that a cancer diagnosis, treatment and the period after treatment can bring.

- Part 1 outlined the uncomfortable thoughts and emotional experiences, such as uncertainty, that being affected by cancer can bring up.

These approaches allow you to face serious difficulties and to experience difficult thoughts and feelings without letting go of what matters most to you. By opening up and allowing yourself to experience difficult thoughts and feelings (while choosing to use strategies that are helpful for you), you can begin to feel more able to cope and to have more time to get on with your life. You can use this time to discover what is meaningful and important to you. This helps you to connect to your values and to live a more fulfilling life, despite all the problems that cancer brings your way.

- Part 2 explored an ACT approach and techniques to help you to reconnect with yourself, your values and a meaningful life, even when you are living with the impact of cancer and difficult thoughts and feelings show up. These were:

  o Dropping anchor and self as context.

  o Defusion or standing back from difficult thoughts.

  o Expansion, acceptance and allowing space for difficult thoughts and feelings.

  o Being compassionate and kind to yourself.

  o Doing what matters to you. Finding and following your values; then committing to take action.

- Part 3 introduced the use of self-care strategies to support your physical and psychological well-being while coping with the impact of cancer. It also gave some practical advice on strategies to manage common problems after cancer: fatigue and pain, eating difficulties and sleep problems. We asked you to consider whether using these strategies could be helpful and keep you on track toward what is important to you.

○ A key message to help you remember these things is to:

Be present, open up, do what works and what matters to you.

Where do I go now? Allowing yourself space to grow

We hope that the skills that you have learned within this book have enabled you to develop a different relationship with your amazing mind: to listen when it is helpful and encouraging you to do things that take you toward a life that you value; to also notice and be kind to yourself when it hooks you in and tries to keep you safe but is unintentionally taking you away from the life you would like to live.

A diagnosis of cancer can be life-changing in many ways. Not all of these are problematic. It can bring to light what really matters to you, enabling you to take control of what you do and to prioritize what is really important to you. You may walk toward a very different life or recognize how much you love the life you already live.

"September 22nd, 2018 marks my 15th anniversary of diagnosis, a life-changing experience which, I believe, has ultimately made me a far more relaxed, tolerant and nicer person. It has taught me so much".

"I may not be one of those people who are climbing mountains to raise money for charity, but I have climbed my own mountain and am living my own life which works for me".

"Now I describe cancer as something that changed me for the better in some ways, something I never thought I'd hear myself saying. I fully understand that's easier for me to say now, 5 years on … still wish it hadn't happened though".

"I am not glad I've had cancer by a long shot, but some positives have come out of it".

Remember you matter

You may have chosen to read parts of the book or you may have read it all. You may choose to come back to parts you missed or dip in and out of it when it feels helpful. Perhaps you read it by yourself or maybe you shared it with your partner, family and friends.

However you choose to use this book, we hope that it has given you a little space to think about what you need right now and what could help you going forward. It might feel now like you have a little more hope that you can be who you want to be, and you are able to find meaning in your life when things are really tough. We hope it also helps you to give yourself permission to look after yourself, maybe just a little bit every day and when you need it most.

When times are tough, you can drop anchor, make some space for what thoughts and feelings have shown up, recognize your skills and strengths and look after yourself.

When things are a little lighter, you can connect, laugh and appreciate or enjoy the small things.

Most of all, we hope that this book helps you to recognize that, despite the cancer, you truly matter and however tough things feel right now, you are not alone.

> "People don't like change, but even difficult change can be good in ways … if you can embrace that and accept that, then you can get through your cancer a lot better … you can give yourself a life that you didn't think you could have in the beginning".

Further reading and resources

Resources for this book

We have created a website to support this book. Within this website, you will find further resources and audio versions of some of the exercises. You can find this website at: www.routledge.com/9780367549244

Below are some resources where you can access information and support for some issues covered in this list. This is just a selection of the resources that are available in the UK. If you would like more detailed information related to your personal needs, please speak with your healthcare team about how to access local services or resources that are available in your area.

ACT and mindfulness books

ACT based

- Harris, R. (2008). The Happiness Trap: How to stop struggling and start living. Boston, MA: Trumpeter.

- Harris, R. (2021). The Reality Slap 2nd Edition: How to survive and thrive when life hits hard. Little, Brown Book Group.

- Harris, R. (2019). ACT Made Simple: An Easy-To-Read Primer on Acceptance and Commitment Therapy (Second Edition). New Harbinger Publications.

- Hayes, S. C. & Smith, S. (2005). Get out of your mind and into your life: The new Acceptance and Commitment Therapy. Oakland, CA: New Harbinger.

- Oliver, J., Hill, J and Morris, E. (2015). ACTivate your life: Using acceptance and mindfulness to build a life that is rich, fulfilling and fun. London, England: Constable & Robinson.

- Owen, R. (2014). Living with the Enemy: Coping with the stress of chronic illness using CBT, mindfulness and acceptance. London: Routledge.

- Owen, R. (2011). Facing the Storm: Using CBT, mindfulness and acceptance to build your resilience when your world's falling apart. London: Routledge.

Mindfulness based

- Burch, V. (2010). Living well with pain and illness: Using mindfulness to free yourself from suffering. London: Piatkus.

- Carlson, L. & Speca, M. (2011). Mindfulness-based cancer recovery. A step-by-step MBSR approach to help you cope with treatment and reclaim your life. New Harbinger Publications.

- Penman, D. & Burch, V. (2013). Mindfulness for Health: A practical guide to relieving pain, reducing stress and restoring wellbeing. London: Piaktus.

- Williams, M. & Penman, D. (2011). Mindfulness: A practical guide to finding peace in a frantic world. London: Piaktus.

Websites

Below are some examples of websites that have some additional resources, exercises and information that you may find useful.

ACT based

The websites below contain free information, resources, videos and exercises based on ACT:

- www.actmindfully.com.au/free-stuff/

- thehappinesstrap.com/free-resources/

- www.getselfhelp.co.uk/act.htm

Mindfulness based

The websites below contain free information, resources, videos and exercises based on mindfulness:

- www.bangor.ac.uk/mindfulness/

- franticworld.com/free-meditations-from-mindfulness/

- www.wyevalley.nhs.uk/services/community-services/pain-management-service/acceptance-and-commitment-therapy-act.aspx

Further self-help

- NHS-based self-help guides: https://web.ntw.nhs.uk/selfhelp/

Apps

Below are some examples of apps that also have some additional resources, exercises and information that you may find useful.

ACT based

● **ACT Companion: The Happiness Trap App**

An ACT-based subscription app designed by Dr. Russ Harris.
www.actcompanion.com/

● **Values Card Sort App**

A free app designed to help you to identify and prioritize your personal values.

Mindfulness based

● **Velindre Mindfulness App**

Guided mindfulness suitable for patients and carers to help you deal with difficult thoughts, feelings and emotions. This app also includes relaxation and guided imagery exercises. The app is free to download and use.
www.velindre-tr.wales.nhs.uk/news/50986

● **Headspace**

An app which teaches you how to meditate and use mindfulness in your everyday life.
www.headspace.com

● **Calm**

An app focusing on sleep and meditation exercises.
www.calm.com

Help with sleep

Sleep Matters
Provides telephone advice and resources concerning sleep problems
www.medicaladvisoryservice.org.uk
020 8994 9874 (each evening 6pm–8pm)

The Sleep Council
Provides helpline, information and resources on improving sleep.
www.sleepcouncil.org.uk
0800 018 7923

Useful resources for sleep

Books

● Espie, C. A. (2012). *Overcoming Insomnia and Sleep Problems: A self-help guide using cognitive behavioural techniques*. London: Constable & Robinson.

Sleep apps

- **Sleepio**

Self-help sleep improvement program and six-week online program.
www.sleepio.com

- **Sleep by Headspace**

Relaxing sleep casts, music and sounds.
www.headspace.com

Health apps

For more health apps, visit the NHS Apps Library:
www.nhs.uk/apps-library/

Cancer-specific information and support

Macmillan Cancer Support
www.macmillan.org.uk
0808 808 00 00
Open seven days a week 8am–8pm
Cancer Research UK
www.cancerresearchuk.org
0808 800 4040
Open Monday–Friday 9am–5pm

Cancer Support UK

www.cancersupportuk.org

There are many other cancer charities that provide information and resources for living with cancer and specific diagnoses.

Information and support for carers

Carers UK
www.carersuk.org

UK Government website
www.gov.uk/carers-uk

In a crisis

If you feel unable to keep yourself safe, the services below will be able to help you:

- Call your GP/GP out-of-hours service.

- Call your local Crisis team if you have the number.

- Go to A&E or call 999 and ask for an ambulance if you unable to travel to A&E.

- Samaritans: Call 116 123 or email jo@samaritans.org (24 hours, 365 days per year).

- Papyrus: Call 0800 068 4141 or email pat@papyrus-uk.org (9am–midnight, 365 days per year).

- Mind: Call 0208 215 2243 or email info@mind.org.uk. www.mind.org.uk/

Flying over thunderstorms metaphor (Delduca and Johnson)

This metaphor has been developed through our work with people affected by cancer, as a way of explaining the core processes of psychological flexibility represented by the ACT Hexaflex (Russ Harris, 2019). It also incorporates some of the other commonly used ACT metaphors and originated from an extension and adaptation of the 'Sky and Weather' and 'Struggle Switch' metaphors (Russ Harris, 2019).

For further information, we have highlighted below how these core processes and metaphors are represented within this metaphor. They are noted in the order they appear in the metaphor:

Element of metaphor	ACT concept
Autopilot mode on	Usual habitual or learned patterns of thinking, responding and behaving
Thinking while flying	Thinking self
Thunderstorm	Thoughts, feelings, sensations and any other painful experiences/sky and weather metaphor
Flying through the thunderstorm (with autopilot on)	Fusion
Criticizing yourself	Overly helpful friend
Noticing the thunderstorm	Contact with present moment
Taking a moment	Pressing pause
Switching autopilot on/off	Struggle switch metaphor
Having choice about what to do	Choice point
Flying through thunderstorm (with autopilot off)	Turning toward the pain/self-compassion
Turning around or landing	Experiential avoidance/away moves
Rising above the thunderstorm	ACT skills: e.g. Defusion, Expansion, Urge Surfing, acceptance and opening up
Watching the weather	Mindfulness/Observer Self
Awareness of bumpy ride/"I'm OK"	Self-compassion
Checking/following your compass	Values
Decision to keep flying in the guided direction	Committed action/Toward moves
Noticing the sky	Self as context/sky and weather metaphor

List of values

Below is a list of some values as ideas for you to consider. It is not an exhaustive list and you may think of others that are relevant to you. You can create your own list, just for you.

You may find it helpful to group the values into three groups:

- Very important to me.

- Important to me.

- Not important to me.

Achievement

Adventure

Authenticity

Authority

Autonomy

Balance

Beauty

Boldness

Care

Challenge

Citizenship

Community

Compassion

Competency

Connection

Contribution

Creativity

Curiosity

Determination

Fairness

Faith

Fame

Friendships

Fun

Growth

Honesty

Humor

Influence

Inner harmony

Justice

Kindness

Knowledge

Leadership

Learning

Love

Loyalty

Meaningful work

Openness

Optimism

Peace

Pleasure

Poise

Popularity

Recognition

Religion

Reputation

Respect

Responsibility

Security

Self-respect

Service

Spirituality

Stability

Status

Success

Trustworthiness

Wealth

Wisdom

Other values

....

....

....

....

....

Index

9780367549244